MOVING FORWARD

The Journey of a Cancer Caregiver

Elmdea Adams

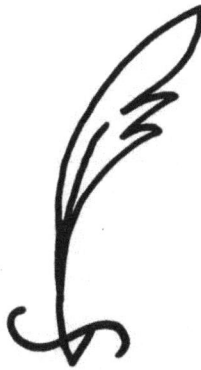

MOVING FORWARD

979-8-218-75502-7 (ebook)

979-8-272-69388-4 (Amazon pbk)

979-8-218-75482-2 (D2D pbk)

This book is a memoir. It is based on the author's notes and recollections of past events and experiences. While the story is true, some names and identifying details have been altered to protect the privacy of individuals. Some events may have been compressed, and dialogue may have been recreated for narrative purposes.

* * *

This book is dedicated to the sixteen members of my
private Facebook group: *Elmdea's Kith & Kin*. More than you can ever
know, your love, understanding, prayers, rituals,
and unwavering support eased my journey of caretaking
and John's death.

Thank you, Anne, Becky, Cathi, Christal, Dana, Donna,
Jenn, Joyce, Kate, Kerrith, Mara, Margi, Sally, Susan,
Suzanne, and Suwaylu from the depths of my heart.

* * *

It is also dedicated to the private Our Wednesday Chats
Zoom group. We've all experienced deep grief
and we are moving forward hand in hand,
sometimes laughing, sometimes crying,
always understanding and supporting each other
as we miss and love our beloveds.

Big hugs (virtual, as usual, lol) to
Marie, Nancy, Pat, and Sandy.

* * *

CONTENTS

OPENING NOTES

What I'm sharing here are my journal entries and social media posts, as well as pertinent comments from friends that were written at the time.

I've included John's social media posts and a few of his emails and texts to give you a small glimpse into who he was and how cancer and its treatments impacted him. I've purposely not used spellcheck or changed any grammar or punctuation in what he wrote. To have done so would diminish the impact of his offerings. He was a wise and gentle man who was a highly respected elder in his communities.

The names of some commenters have been changed, some have not. All of the doctor's names have been changed.

It's taken five years, four months, two weeks, and six days from the date of John's diagnosis for this book to reach completion. I thought I'd publish it within two years of John's death, but realized I couldn't emotionally handle re-reading everything. It's been a process of patience, love, and trust. It's the completion of a promise I made to myself to honor the pain and grief that John and I experienced. This book is a compassionate gift from John and me to caretakers and those with cancer, and late stage esophageal cancer in particular. You aren't alone in your journey, much as it feels that way. It's my hope that this book provides insights to those of you supporting caregivers and the grieving.

It never occurred to me to get a second opinion. John was so sure, and it wasn't my life or my decision. I was in shock and things were moving too quickly.

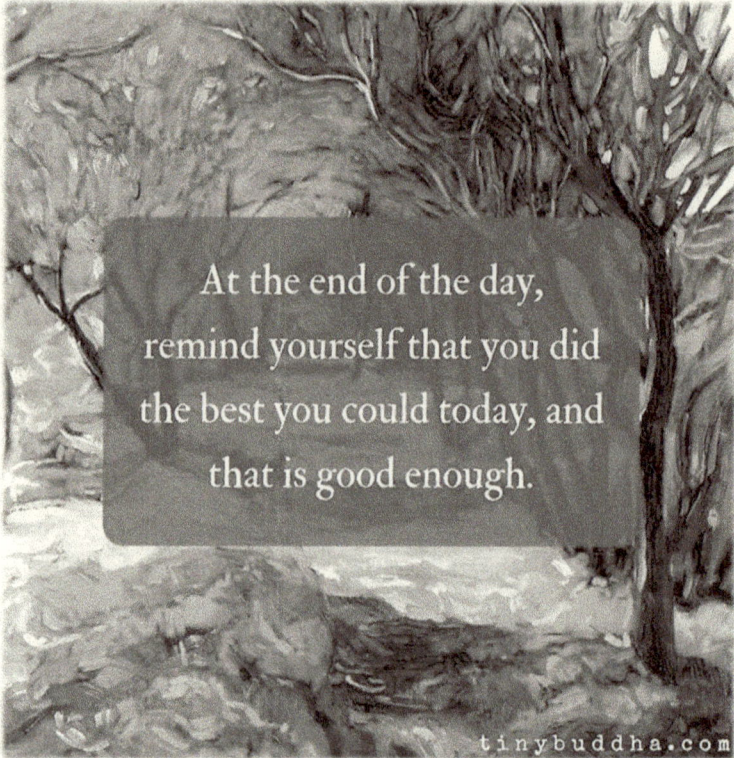

At the end of the day, remind yourself that you did the best you could today, and that is good enough.

tinybuddha.com

PART I:
OUR BEGINNINGS

John and I first connected sometime in the early 2000's. I was single and I wanted to know where my partner, my love, was and why he wasn't in my life yet. I was meditating and I asked. I heard a voice in my head. He said he was John and that we both had things to learn and work out before we could get together.

Pfffft. That was NOT the answer I wanted. I wasn't interested in more waiting, so I joined Match.com. Interesting enough guys, mostly, but not anyone who survived the first careful date or two. I left Match and continued my mostly happy single life, dating here and there. At some point, I decided I'd give Match another go. Again, the same "thanks but no thanks". I was ready to cancel again when one of those "you might also consider" profiles showed up. He looked kinda interesting. Nothing left to lose by getting in touch.

We exchanged the usual anonymous Match.com protected e-mails. He actually sounded interesting. We exchanged a few more.

He suggested we get together for an "inspection dinner" (his term, lol).

I figured why not? If nothing else, I'd have a good meal. We set the time and place for the following week. I can't remember what came up, but it was something with girlfriends, so I rescheduled it. NOT what you're supposed to do. He was fine with it.

Here are a few of our emails before we met in person.

* * *

Subject: We'll see if my magic decoder ring worked
From: John
Date: Thu, Aug 26, 2010, at 11:02 PM
Hi Elmdea,

Hmmm… hopefully the Lord of the Northern Elementals is feeling benevolent. ;-) Not one icicle on the house today! It's actually going to let me take my daughter to the Jefferson County fair on Sat., which will be good. She usually calls me up at 7 pm on a weekend night and asks me if I want to hang out. The concept of planning has not entered her vocabulary yet.

I move around with music too, but I'm always returning to the old Celtic stuff, especially the slow airs. I have the DVD of that Alhambra concert, but I've been saving it for when the weather gets cool.

I like bluegrass, reggae, some jazz and old 60s/70s stuff. I'll listen to one thing for a while and then drift off to something else. Reggae is the bomb for straightening up the house!

I know what you mean about sitting around with the "youngsters" — It really made me laugh a couple of years ago when I was teaching at Shepherd and I heard some of my students talking about "that old guy."

In my office we have a senior or greybeard wing and a 30's wing.

Did you see the full moon last night? I went out and sat on the porch for a while before bed. The clouds were gorgeous.

Looks like the turnout for the drum circle tomorrow will be good. It's really nice when the drumming dancing and the fire all fall into synch — it's transporting. I'm looking forward to it.

Hope you have a great day tomorrow.

BB
John

* * *

From: Elmdea
Date: Fri, Aug 27, 2010, at 4:58 PM
John,

    Your decoder ring worked just fine! And happy to hear there aren't any icicles in the offing.

    I saw the moon last night, sat outside in it's beautiful light, listening to the crickets.

    Had an amazing regression session with someone today — they spent most of their time in the between lives space, interacting with their guides. Amazing… I'm so blessed to be doing this work!

    I'm fairly eclectic music-wise. Exceptions are hip-hop and rap, and a little bit of country goes a long, long way. Mostly, though, I don't have anything on. I tend to live in silence.

    Have a great time at your drumming circle tonight!!!
Blessings,
Elmdea

* * *

From: John
Date: Fri, Aug 27, 2010, at 5:41 PM
Hi Elmdea,

    Interestingz, I tend to live in silence as well. That was always my inclination, then a few years back I lost most of the hearing in my right ear. It's gotten a little better, but the music has to be pretty loud (or headphones). Little memory bubble popped about Paul Winter and all the years I listened to his stuff. IMHO rap and hip hop ain't music — just children with expensive recording equipment :)

    Do you like to sing? I can't sing very well but I've been going to a sacred harp singing group in Berryville for about 20 years. It is really powerful music. They meet about 8 or 9 times a year. I went to a wonderful two day sing with them in Winchester over the summer. It was at the historic Miller house next to the Thai place in Old Town. People from all over the east coast came.

I'm looking forward to hearing about your work — it's something I've brushed up against, but have never really known anyone who was deeply involved. I have done some shamanic trance work, and it was pretty interesting.

I'm hopeful that we get a good turnout tonight. The weather has finally cooled off so that having a fire isn't an act of lunacy. We did it in July when it was 100. I'll drum you a tune and ricochet it off the moon!
BB
John

* * *

From: Elmdea
Date: Sat, Aug 28, 2010 at 5:02 PM
John,

Sorry to take so long to respond — busy day today and so I'll write more later. Looking forward to meeting you "face to face" tomorrow!
Elmdea

* * *

From: Elmdea
Date: Sat, Aug 28, 2010 at 11:26 PM
John,

I'd forgotten about Paul Winter. One of my favorites was Taj Mahal. Thank you for sharing and reconnecting me with his music!

I do sing. Used to play guitar and sing — even had a paying gig once. I learned, very quickly, that that was NOT my thing. My genre was folk music.

How was the day with your daughter? I ended up going to the Luckett's Fair with a friend and a friend of hers. Let's just say I've had better and more enjoyable experiences. Twilight Polo in Warrenton was good — just stayed for part of the first game and touched base with a bunch of folks I know. Then Beth and I went and got a bite to eat in Warrenton and then over to her place to just hang out a bit.

The Census Bureau has officially terminated me for Lack of Work and sent me the paperwork to go apply for unemployment. I'm finding that I'm actually feeling relieved. It was a great experience and I'm glad it's done. It was a sort of whip-saw experience and it would take me at least a week to get my feet back under me after each operation (there were 3 of them). Now I can settle back into my work with fresh eyes and fresh energy.

See ya soon (and thank you for the energy ricochet off the moon!!!)
Elmdea

* * *

From: John
Date: Sun, Aug 29, 2010, at 10:10 AM
Hi Elmdea,

Drum circle was great — we had 2 new people show up and they were both neat. Got some good drumming in and broke at 11. Had fun with my daughter — county fairs are just so .. salt of the earth. Saw the tractor pull, ate hot dogs and funnel cake, listened to some good bluegrass and wandered around the midway. I love watching the people. I'm worried I may be having too much fun this weekend… and it's far from over :)

I loved Taj Mahal too. Saw him a couple of times in the 70s (yikes!). He was so smooth. He's still around… :)

I'm impressed that you had a paying gig. Closest I ever came to that was singing folk songs for beer money with a friend outside a bar in Lawrence, Ks. We were asked to go away.

Looking forward to seeing you!
John

* * *

Sunday, August 29, 2010

We got together for our "inspection dinner", meeting in the town square near the restaurant where we'd be having dinner. I looked at him from a distance and thought "Well, a free dinner. He looks really old, too many wrinkles, and overweight. Not the kind of guy I'm looking for."

Twenty minutes into dinner, I realized something else was going on. This felt different.

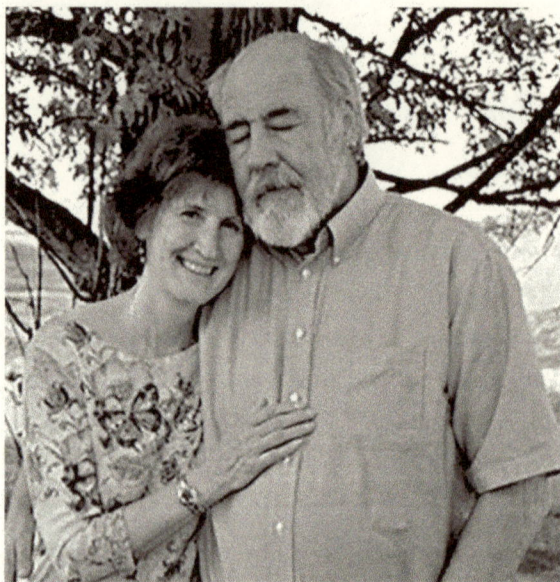

John and Elmdea, 2010

We ended up sitting on a bench in the park, talking for another three hours. We were both sharing things you don't usually share until you've known someone for months or years. He walked me to my car and gave me a kiss on my cheek and said he'd be in touch.

On my way home, I nearly ran a red light. When it happened a second time, I knew I was in altered consciousness and needed to really pay attention. I opened the windows so the air was moving around me.

Monday, August 30, 2010

John told me today that he'd taken the wrong road west, making a normal one hour trip two hours.

We agreed that there was something else going on here. There was.

To paraphrase a quote from somewhere, we are re-learning the songs of each other's hearts and singing them to each other because we've forgotten them in all these years in this incarnation.

Wednesday, October 6, 2010

It's been an intense month or so. I met my soul love, John, at the end of August. On September 10, my father died. On the 13th, John and I went to New York for a druid gathering. I could feel the protective energy bowl that had been put up over the camp.

A few days ago, I sat on my back porch steps, meditating and seeing if I could reach my father's spirit. I did. Took me totally by surprise.

He was pumping his arms up and down saying "I did it! I did it!"

"Did what?" I asked.

"Lived exactly the kind of life I'd planned so I'd have exactly the experiences I wanted to."

By the end of our conversation, I was able to honestly thank my father for how he helped shape me into the person I am. He was a bigot, a misogynist, an alcoholic. What I've taken away from that is that, no matter how messy someone's life looks from the outside, they may be exactly on track for what their soul wants to experience in this life.

Saturday, October 9, 2010

John and I spent another wonderful day at his house up in the West Virginia hills. I feel so relaxed, so at peace, when I'm here. The house is on the top of a ridge, with no close neighbors. It's just so quiet. I love the dragon flags he's hung between the posts of the front porch!

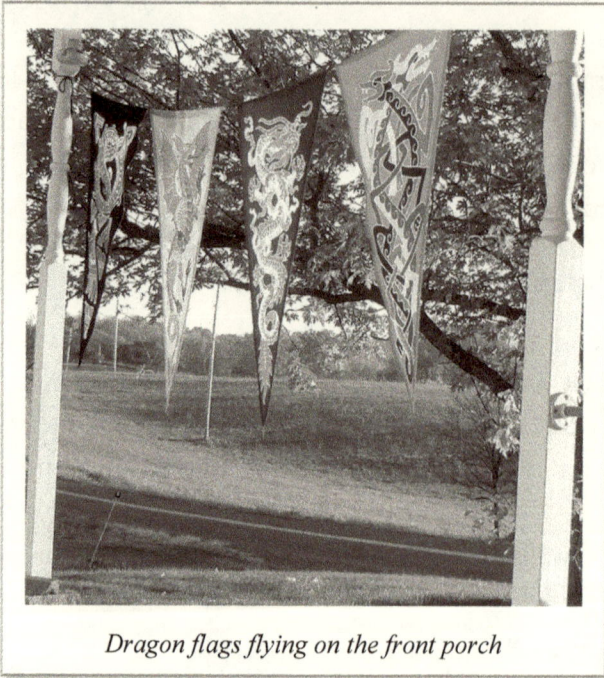

Dragon flags flying on the front porch

Sunday, November 21, 2010

Gorgeous day here – based on the weather forecast, this may be one of the last semi-warm days for quite a while!! There is a sweet chorus of birds and the light has that luminous fall quality. Time for a walk (with my darling John), to be IN the woods, WITH the birds.

I'm grateful for the walking path behind my condo. I found a seven foot long branch that's been shaped by vines. It needs to sit for a year or so but it will make a beautiful staff.

Friday, November 29, 2010

It's been a lovely long weekend at the beach, at John's dad's beach house in Lewes. Last night, there was a 15 mile back-up on I-70 going into Baltimore/Washington, D.C. Soooo grateful we were going the OTHER direction!!

Friday, December 10, 2010

John proposed tonight. I said yes! It's been both scary and amazing. And it feels beyond right.

I suspect my sister and a good number of my friends are going to question the wisdom of this. We've only known each other a little more than three months. And we've known each other for much longer. I had a "vision" sometime in these past months. It was a series of quick snapshots in my mind, each of a different life John and I have shared. We've done this life dance many times. We waited until later in this life to re-connect and move forward together.

Sunday, December 19, 2010

I'm feeling very loved. John is fixing us spaghetti and homemade meatballs (he's making them!), with salad and garlic bread for dinner tonight. Yummmmm!!

Wednesday, December 29, 2010

John invited me to celebrate his birthday with him. He had already purchased a ticket for a ten-day Caribbean cruise for himself because he never liked that his birthday was in the middle of cold, snowy winter. I accepted the gift. He's purchasing a second ticket for me. It will be a sort of trial run of how well we get along together while traveling and in close quarters. Not everyone is good travel company, let alone living together company.

Monday, February 7 – Tuesday, February 18, 2011

We had a wonderful time on our cruise, made some good friends, and just enjoyed the warmth and being away from winter. Close quarters wasn't an issue and we had fun just being together. I love that man.

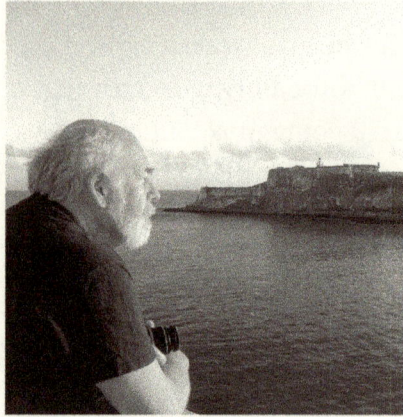

John, enjoying morning coffee as we cruise past El Morro in Old San Juan, Puerto Rico, 2011

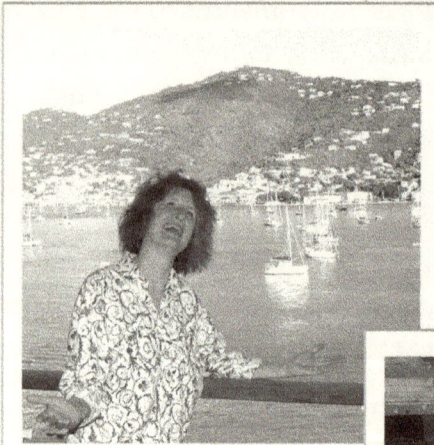

Elmdea, at St. Thomas harbor, 2011

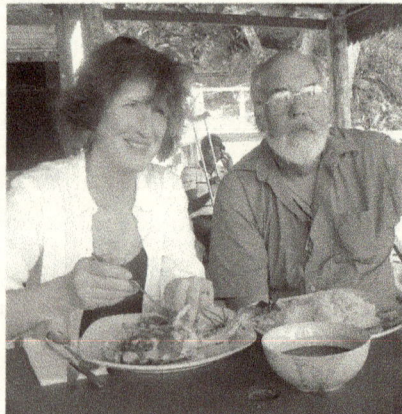

Enjoying fresh caught fish, Samana, Dominican Republic, 2011

Saturday, April 2, 2011

Today I moved. I'm now a West Virginia woman. So many boxes to unpack and then find room for everything. And it's all good. It feels so right to be here, with John, knowing I don't have to leave to go home again. I'm home now, here, with him.

Friday, May 6, 2011

John called to me to come to the front porch quick. A rainbow. Right there across the road, so bright against the storm darkened sky. We just watched until it faded, feeling blessed. It's the first one we've seen together up here.

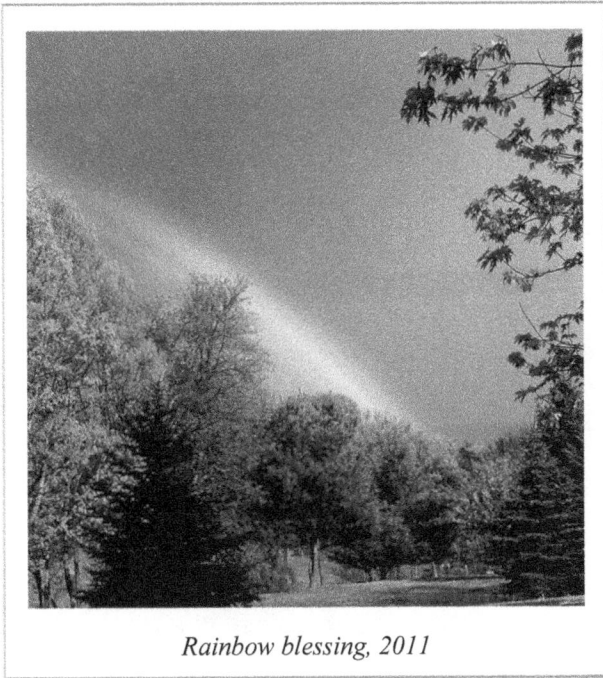

Rainbow blessing, 2011

Sunday, May 15, 2011

Today, a dear friend and Druid Priestess handfasted John and me in the presence of a few friends.

"Make no mistake – you will be bound together, through this life and those following, whether you stay together in this life or not."

John and I both feel this and celebrate the rightness of our bond of love, respect, and partnership. A friend told us he wasn't sure he'd ever seen anyone look at each other quite like we did.

This is our true marriage, in our hearts. Next weekend we'll have a traditional wedding

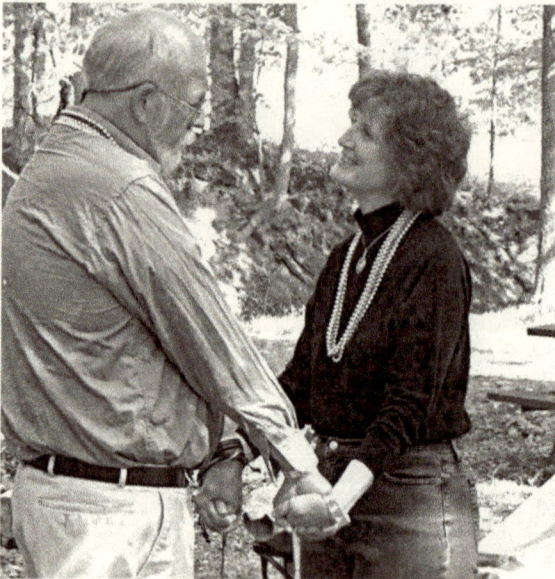

John and Elmdea
Handfasting, 2011

Saturday, May 21, 2011

Today, my good and dear friend Suwaylu married John and I in the presence of his family and mine, as well as many friends. As requested, people brought food to share as their wedding present. It was a beautiful and affirming celebration.

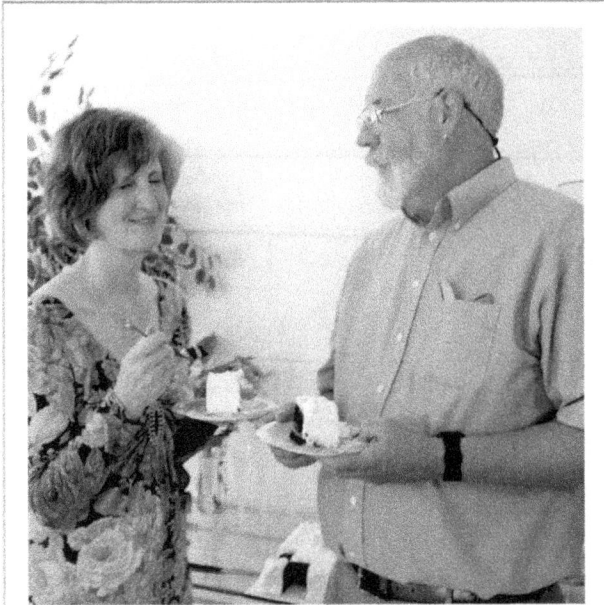

Getting ready to feed each other pieces of the wedding cake, 2011

It did feel odd to take our wedding rings off. We've been wearing them since last Saturday and they got to be blessed again. It feels like an affirmation of our commitment and love to and for each other.

Friday, November 25, 2011

What an amazing day! First the book festival, then John took me out for dinner, and then BACK to the MAC Ice House for the Roots Music Concert – local bluegrass and rock-a-billy music – multi-generation, multi-family groups playing absolutely first-class music. I am blessed to be living in this community! We both loved it and I'm looking forward to more concerts.

Saturday, December 17, 2011

John took me out to dinner tonight. Got called "miss" by the server. I can't remember the last time that happened. It was fun. The homemade coconut cake for dessert… well… remember that scene from *When Harry Met Sally* and the other diner said "I want what she has."? That cake was that good. OMG!!!

April 6, 2011

This popped up on my timeline this morning, as I recreate my life in partnership with John. Old patterns and new choices being seen. What richness!! It's wonderful. John and I are both committed to our individual growth and our growth as partners. It's a lovely (and loving) synergy and flow!!

> *"Don't grieve. Anything you lose comes around in another form. The child weaned from mother's milk now drinks wine and honey mixed."*
> ~ *Rumi*

March 22, 2012

John: Turkeys were out before dawn… mist spun their gobbling round and round.

* * *

And so our lives progressed as we continued to learn more and more about each other, appreciating the wonder and beauty of how we both complement and match each other. There was always something new to learn about John, not because he was hiding anything, but because of the depth of who he was and his years of experiences. I know he found the same with me.

In 2014 and 2016 I had some medical issues, some more serious than others and all treatable and treated. John was there for me through it all, holding my hand, reassuring me, loving me.

Looking Back

My only regret is that I didn't fully realize how precious the ordinary, everyday moments are: having dinner as usual, the smell of John's morning coffee, John making up stories and roaring with laughter when I finally caught on, quick hugs, waving at him sitting on the front porch as I drove into town, and watching him play one of his on-line games when I came into our shared office. Seeing John's ritual before he went to sleep: lying on his left side propped up on his elbow, left hand keeping his book open, and Miz Alice kitty keeping him company as he munched a blueberry turnover.

And yet, until those ordinary everyday kinds of moments began to disappear, there was no way for me to fully realize how very precious they really were.

PART II:
ILL HEALTH

Monday, July 30, 2018

On July 20th, I had back surgery to remove a piece of herniated disc that was lodged against my sciatic nerve for seven months. I couldn't drive, between the pain and the Percocet I needed to control it. The surgery wasn't the instant fix I'd hoped it would be. I'm learning what the nurse meant when she said nerves can take up to two years to heal.

Tuesday, October 2, 2018

John saw his GP today for his regular six month check-up. There wasn't anything remarkable per the doctor. But I have my doubts. I feel like John isn't telling me something, perhaps to protect me, since I'm still recovering from my back surgery in July. It just doesn't seem like John is eating as much.

Sunday, October 28, 2018

John isn't eating as much as he used to. I make the same amount of food as I always have and there's more left over. I don't want to pester him, but something isn't right. He's always been hungry, always munching on something like cheese sticks, except he isn't eating as many now. I don't think he's replaced it with something else. I do most of the food shopping, so I'd know.

He loves his Diet Coke, drinking four or five a day. He's drinking three or four a day now. Not a big change, but still. It all has me wondering.

I've got my doubts about how good his GP is. Time will tell.

Thursday, November 22, 2018

I fixed us Cornish Game hens for Thanksgiving today since neither of us much like turkey. John took two bites of his, then excused himself in a hurry and went into the bathroom. I could hear him trying to vomit. When he came back to the table, he said it wasn't the food. He was just having problems swallowing every now and then. He asked me to put his dinner away because he just wasn't hungry anymore.

Wednesday, November 28, 2018

He visited his doctor, who said everything looked fine, although John had lost some weight.

We know something is wrong and we're thinking maybe a hernia. At the outside, Barrett's Esophagus.

Tuesday, December 4, 2018

John saw his doctor again today and it was agreed he needed to see a Gastroenterologist. I'm relieved something is finally getting done.

Friday, December 14, 2018.

I'm sooooo unimpressed with John's GP. They'd been very slow getting the appointment set up (a week) and then it was with a medical group that didn't accept our insurance. John let them know.

Today, his GP's office called quite pleased with themselves. They'd found someone who could see John in April.

I said "John, I'm making an appointment for you with my GP, Dr. Grant." John nodded yes.

Monday, December 17, 2018

We saw Dr. Grant today. He was very concerned and had his staff start immediately with getting John referred and scheduled for a barium swallow.

Saturday, December 22, 2018

I'm starting to get concerned. John couldn't do the barium swallow yesterday (he literally couldn't swallow the liquid), so he was scheduled for a CT scan today. It showed "something of concern."

Sunday, December 30, 2018

John's endoscopy is scheduled for Wednesday, January 2. Thank God! We can find out what's really going on. He's lost about 14 pounds in three to four months. He weighed 277 pounds in early October. In early December, he weighed 263. He can only eat liquids now. His barium swallow showed his lower esophagus is 2 or 3 mm wide, about the size of a pencil – not very!

I've been thinking I've been doing well, and had some anxiety stuff last night. Hmmm. Guess not. At least I seem to be catching myself earlier.

I just don't have a good feeling about this. But I don't know how much of that is intuitive and how much is catastrophizing. I find myself "playing" at "I live alone, without John." It's good and it's bad. If it's as bad as I'm afraid it will be, the grief will be way more than I'm willing to acknowledge right now. Which is reasonable. We don't have enough information yet.

John just "feels different" – like he's almost not here? Shifted somewhere? It could well be his own way of dealing with this. He really, really doesn't like change and he's got that blasted "I'm strong, I'm man, I'm not weak/vulnerable/scared" thing going on.

I'm grateful I have Margi, my therapist, to work with on this. I see her on Thursday.

Monday, December 31, 2018

John

> *So I got my dad and his GF some xmas presents which were delivered on 12/11/18. Little stuff iPad case and a book reading stand. I asked them if they had arrived, and they said no.*
>
> *I checked delivery info to make sure — they live in an apt complex, so things go missing. I reordered another set which got there today. My dad said they were exactly the same as the presents he had gotten for his GF.*
>
> *<I scratch my head??> Later on he mentioned that he didn't remember ordering anything.*
>
> *When I got off the phone with him I was giggling. What happened is my first set arrived and he gave it to GF. She assumed he had ordered it for her and was happy.*
>
> *My dad is 96. I'm keeping my mouth shut.*

Tuesday, January 22, 2019

John may have esophageal cancer. A PET scan is being ordered and the biopsy's done. They tried to put in a stent yesterday in Baltimore. It wouldn't fit. So we wait and John remains on his liquid, highly pureed diet. He's lost 66 pounds since the beginning of October. That's only 3½ months.

Looking Back

While we both knew something was going on, neither of us suspected cancer. We had thought maybe a hiatal hernia or, at worst, Barrett's esophagus. Cancer never entered our minds, or at least mine. I have no idea if it had entered John's.

We were in shock. We stood by each other as we always had. We did a fairly good job of taking it one day at a time.

And we were human: scared, sometimes in tears, holding each other, and discovering humor was still alive and well.

PART III:
KITH & KIN

Thursday, January 24, 2019

I've decided to set up a private social media support group of close friends and family for myself. I need to be able to share what's happening easily and quickly. I'm calling it *Elmdea's Kith & Kin*. I anticipate I'll need a place where I can safely share what I'm going through and ask for support.

Posting on my public page isn't an option. I don't want all kinds of advice from all kinds of people. It's too much to keep track of and deal with. There are sixteen people I'll be inviting to join. John isn't part of this group, by choice, and by his agreement.

I need to be able to rant, worry, vent, cry, and who knows what else that John won't be able to see. I need that space to ensure I can be present to John's needs, without projecting (too many) of mine on him.

I suspect I'm really going to need that space and that support.

Friday, January 25, 2019

Kate posted some pics earlier this week of a vintage rug loom her elderly neighbor is selling. Just looking at it made me happy. I went over today to look at it and I bought it. Now to figure out how to get it home. It was her husband's, and he'd inherited it from his father, who had bought it new. An old Union 36 Rug Loom.

By the time I got home, John had heard from Dr. Grant. John has esophageal cancer. We're now waiting to get a PET to see if/where it has/hasn't spread.

Saturday, January 26, 2019

It's an "interesting" experience. Yesterday was calm and felt like before all this started, until we got the news from Dr. Grant. Today, not so much. Almost in tears a number of times. John didn't do his usual routine with taking his meds and he had erps all day. It's so hard to watch (and listen to), knowing there is nothing, nada, zero I can do to help.

The good news today was I got some leads on how to take the loom apart to move it, so I can tell my moving guy what needs to be done! And John had a dream about the loom last night. It had us both smiling.

Monday, January 28, 2019

Aaaand… my rug loom is home. So glad I hired some moving/handy people to do it. Not sure what her name is yet, but I know she'll let me know. Now to weave a rug, or two or three. I basically see this as a meditative thing for me to do.

Tuesday, January 29, 2019

Success! The PET scan is scheduled for this coming Friday at 10 at Robinwood in Hagerstown and… he's on the waitlist. It won't be Wednesday as we'd hoped cuz their machine is down for routine maintenance that day. But we're both relieved. Progress is happening.

The PET scan will take anywhere from 2-3 hours, between the injection (45-60 minutes for it to be fully in his system) and the scan (1 to 1½ hours).

John informs me that the cafeteria has really good hamburgers (they've been on his mind a LOT lately) and (he said as an aside) "they have your kind of stuff too". Which means salads and veggie kinds of things.

John claims he was born hungry. I can believe it. Now, he literally can't swallow his food, even if he chews it and chews it.

It has to be totally pulverized in the blender with some liquid and then he takes bitty sips. He can manage about 1/3 cup and then has to stop so it can move thru the constriction. If he tries to hurry it, it comes back up with lots of mucus for hours, literally.

Friday, February 1, 2019

Today was John's PET scan in Hagerstown to find out if the cancer is contained or if its spread. And today it's snowing.

I normally don't venture out on days like this, but this Had. To. Be. Done!

Three cheers for growing up in Colorado and learning how to drive in the snow. Those early lessons stay. And... the idiot drivers seem to have stayed home.

Now to wait for the results.

Tuesday, February 5, 2019

No news re: the results of John's PET scan yet. He's thinking Friday, I'm hoping sooner. This hold and wait is hard. The loom is helping. I hope all of you like rag rugs cuz I'm going to have plenty!

Thursday, February 7, 2019

I'm sitting here with tears rolling down my face. Just heard from the doctor. John's cancer is definitely Stage 3 (it's spread to some lymph nodes). It might be Stage 4 (there's a spot in his lung they aren't sure about, but it might be cancer). We're being referred to a different team in Baltimore who we should hear from by Monday for an appointment to get treatment going. At this point, it will be radiation/chemo before surgery to remove the tumor.

I'm letting myself be all weepy, alone, until I'm not. I just have to. I can't keep it in. And I don't want John worrying about me. His worries are so much more than mine.

Friday, February 8, 2019

I'm doing better this morning and so is John. I absolutely know that the love all you here in my Kith and Kin group are sending is helping.

John and I know it'll be up and down and we're focusing on today, which is a good day. We've no real idea of what's coming and I can already tell that having that on-line support group is going to be a sanity and heart saver for me. I'm crying grateful tears for the people who support and love me.

* * *

John heard from the doctor in Baltimore today. We're meeting with the multidisciplinary team (we'll find out exactly what that means when we get there) next Friday, the 15th at 2. They only meet on Fridays so that was the soonest appointment.

The next day (the 16th) is John's birthday.

We're grateful we're getting in as soon as that. We both suspect things will pick up speed after that.

Saturday, February 9, 2019

Turns out we're going to one of the better places in the country to treat John's kind of cancer. I'm amazed at how many people/disciplines come together for this. I suspect we'll be getting to know some of these folks very well.

It's making a difference, mentally and emotionally, for us to know we'll be working with people who are among the best in the country!

* * *

Tomorrow is a different sort of big day. John's father (who will be 97 in a couple of weeks) and his partner, Ero (who is 82) are coming out to see John. Ero's daughter is driving them out from Washington D.C. John is an only child.

His dad hasn't been super healthy lately, so it's even more important. They'll be here about noon and I'm "fixing" a grazing sort of lunch: sandwich makings. Our thought is it will make it easier for John and his dad to have some time on their own, while Ero, Mara, and I chat and... maybe I show them my loom?

On the self-care front, I went to a thrift store yesterday. It was $5 a bag day. Scrubs, flannel jammie pants, sheets, curtains, and tops. I got the ties cuz I saw something in the Sakiori Japanese weaving book that looked really interesting... after I get a little better at this weaving thing. I've got lots of cutting and sewing-strips-together opportunities. That stills my mind.

The ties don't have food spots on 'em! I'll be collecting ties for a bit to have enough to do...? I'll be checking out other thrift stores too.

Sunday, February 10, 2019

John's a little nervous this morning, but looking forward to it. I'm feeling pretty relaxed, especially compared to how I used to be: everything needing to be perfect. Yay for learning to relax around that!

* * *

It was an absolutely wonderful visit! We pretty much left John and his dad alone in the living room while we (me, Ero, Mara, and Mara's boyfriend David) hung out in the kitchen/dining room or the 2nd porch aka loom room. It was a very loving visit all around. John was/is grateful to have had that time with his father.

John and his Dad, 2019

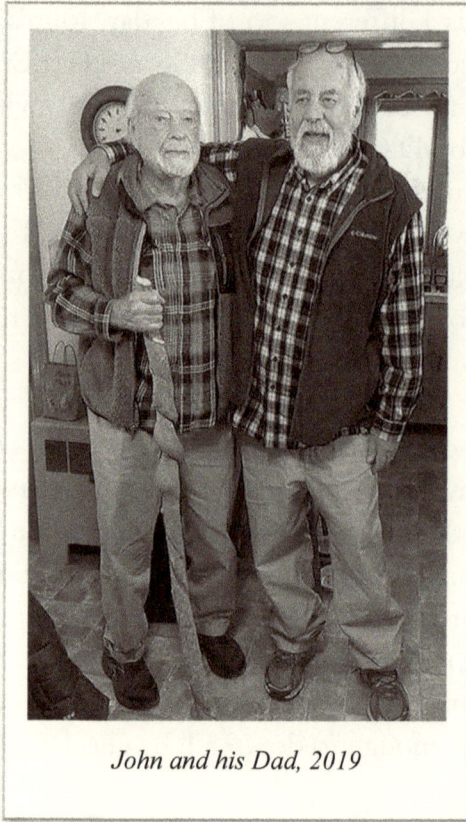

One of the lovely things that happened was John and I gave Mara the staff we made from the heavy vine sculpted branch we found in November of 2010, soon after we'd met. Mara loved it. And so did John Sr.

Monday, February 11, 2019

A wonderful and beautiful thing happened today. John set aside his pride (a HUGE letting go) and asked his friends for help. He's setting up his own private FB group: *Planning For John's 70th Birthday Party*.

John wants me in his group. I asked why and he just shrugged. Looking at who the members are of each group, I've realized how different their focuses are. This one is for support as I navigate caring for both me and for John, making sure I do good self-care. John's is about support in healing and navigating the rough physical and emotional road ahead of him.

In many ways, it still doesn't feel real to me. I'm appreciating this time because I know it will soon be very real as he begins treatment. Thank you again for being here for me now and as this unfolds.

Monday, February 11, 2019

John on his social media page:

I'm going to be needing a little help from my friends.

I am asking my friends for their prayers, healing energy and support.

Long story short, I had what I thought was acid reflux which kept getting worse. Couldn't swallow and have lost a lot of weight. I am now diagnosed with esophageal cancer. I am grateful I have been accepted as a patient at the University of Maryland Cancer Center in Baltimore. I am going there on Friday to discuss treatment options.

The whole experience has been surreal. I haven't felt sick, just weak from not being able to eat. I have been living on protein shakes, jello, etc., for about 3 months, but really not being able to get enough calories to stop my weight loss. I would wrestle a pack of bears for a cheeseburger.

I am likely looking at the whole nine yards treatment wise – chemo, radiation, and surgery. I know that will be rugged. My hearth gods have strongly suggested that I set my pride aside and reach out to as many of my friends as I can because I have many wise friends. I have very good support from my family and local friends, but I'm going need all the support I can get.

I have set up a private FB group for anyone who is interested in coming along for the ride. PM me if you're interested.

* * *

Many thanks to all who responded to my posts! Right now I'm sort of in holding pattern waiting until I go to Baltimore on Friday to find out what is next. It is good to have friends by my side :)

Wednesday, February 13, 2019

John to his group

Been thinking today about feeling old and vulnerable. I've enjoyed pretty good health most of my life and have always been physically strong. Not so much these day. The tumor has largely blocked my esophagus and some days I can swallow limited amounts of protein shakes, cream of wheat, etc. Other days not much goes down except water and jello type things. I haven't been able to eat "real food" (anything that won't go through a pretty fine strainer) for months.

Not getting enough to eat for a long time makes you crazy. I see a truck with cheeseburgers on the side and want to hijack it. I want to rob a chinese restaurant and steal all the food. I get cravings for stuff that I really never liked and haven't eaten in years. Kind of like the stories about shipwrecked sailors.

This particular issue will be fixed. I have already had two endoscopies and one attempt to put a stent in. I am going to be very clear when I meet with the doctors Friday that I am probably marginal for chemo and radiation unless my nutrition comes way up. Choices are a stent opening up my esophagus, a stomach feeding tube, or a tube into my lower intestine. My research shows me that when chemo and radiation are done, I'm looking at major surgery to get rid of the bad stuff and hook up the good stuff, and that some kind of feeding tupe will be required. But that's done the road a bit.

So being physically weak makes me feel vulnerable, No real surprise there. My body image is usually a few years back – I'm really not that old – 69 on Saturday – but I guess that I had hoped that my "major life adventures involving shitty stuff" were done. Been through a few of those and survived. The path set by the Gods doesn't have to make sense to me. I just need to do what I can do to effect the present and influence the weave.

Right now I'm just waiting for things to unfold. Thanks for a place where I can just let stuff out without worrying about getting it right .

A reconstruction of my esophagus is what I'm looking at after they neutralize the "chaos energy" causing the problem.

Elmdea is being a huge help getting me through this.

Thursday, February 14, 2019

It's been a quiet week for me. I still feel pretty centered. We leave about 11:30 tomorrow for our appointment at 2 in Baltimore. It's scheduled for an hour. John and I both have questions (which will probably be answered before we ask them). Not much else we can do to prepare.

I've got John's med list done and he's writing up his Quality of Life "things". I suspect top of his list is enough food to actually feed his body's needs. What has been hard is knowing how little he's been eating because it just won't go thru that tiny opening.

He's scared. I sooooo understand that. If nothing else, all my medical issues these past few years have granted me greater empathy.

I think I've been purposely not thinking about what they'll be sharing, suggesting, saying so I can stay focused and not freak out too much.

I discovered yesterday that there's an easy "record" utility in my phone! I'm taking notes AND I'm going to record it.

In other news, I'm scheduled for my next Transforaminal injection for my back next Wednesday. It also turns out that WxRisk.com is saying there's a strong possibility of an ice storm Tues/Wed. He's rarely wrong.

The pain doctor's office is in Winchester, an hour away. I've made a backup appointment. March 13, three weeks away, was the soonest opening they had. I'm also on their wait list. I really don't want to have to wait that long.

It's been seven months since my discectomy surgery and my sciatic nerve root is still healing and it still hurts. Not as bad as it did, but it hurts.

So there's that on my plate as well. All I know to do is trust the process.

Friday, February 15, 2019

We're here! Traffic was a breeze. The cancer center has a separate check in and the waiting area is actually nice.

They just called John back to "take vitals".

* * *

We just got home (7 pm) . We were there for 2 hours, with lots of wait time and talking to one doctor. For about an hour.

The news is not good. Dr. Jafra thinks it's Stage 4 because the spot in his lung has grown since the CT scan 2 months ago. There's also a suspicious spot on T12 in his mid-back. John will be getting an MRI to get more information on that.

The only doctor who saw us was the medical oncologist (Dr. Jafra). And there's no gene therapy or immunotherapy for esophageal cancer. John is choosing to go for the chemo that's available. It will start in about 2 weeks after they put the port in. They'll also do a biopsy on his lung at that point, with a long needle.

When the doctor recommended chemo, John immediately said yes, then turned to me and said "I know it's not what you'd choose. It's what I need to do." I nodded and reached for his hand. He could tell I was near tears.

Radiation and surgery to remove the cancer aren't an option. He'll talk to the gastro doc to see if a stent can be put in.

I'm emotionally and physically wiped out right now. I drove 5 hours today and held it together cuz driving while crying isn't recommended.

John is much more accepting of all this than I am. And I can feel the shift in him. I don't have words for it, I just feel it.

Friday, February 15, 2019

John to his group:

Went up to the U Md in Balt today to meet with the treatment people. Staff was nice but the news was not. They went over my petscan and found, in addition to one or two funky lymphodes (which I already knew about and which put me at stage 3) , a glowy spot in my right lung and a glowy spot on my spine. Tests will be done on the lung and spine. If they are cancerous, then I am at Stage 4 metastisis and basically only eligible for chemo at this time. I will be starting chemo in the next two weeks. They are going to schedule one appointment to put in the port for the chemo and start and do a biopsy on my lung.

None of this was welcome news. Looks like it will be up to chemo, the will of the gods, my genes, and the support of my family and friends.

Thanks you all for your continued energy and prayers.

In the adding insult to injury dept – we are 1 hour deep with Dr. Jafra – and the nurse comes in and says my insurance company is saying they are not going to cover it. WTF I had a procedure on the 3rd floor of the same hospital 3 weeks ago and there were not any issues. Turns out the cancer center on the first floor was technically a different entity than the rest of the hospital and it ended up ok, after a lot of staff work on their part. The insurance company's authorization policy consists mainly of putting people on hold and hoping you will go away.

So a big tip of the hat to all the support staff that has been helping me get insurance company stupidity resolved throughout my adventure!

Saturday, February 16, 2019

I got some much needed sleep last night. And it still feels very unreal. I may be in shock. Whole new territory.

We're navigating this together. We're making plans on next steps. I'm sensing this may be some of our deepest and best times together.

Aaaaaand – it's Stage 4. We went to Baltimore yesterday to meet with a cancer team. We only met the medical oncologist.

The spot in John's lung is "active" and grown since his CT scan on December 22. He also has a spot on T12 in his spine.

John will start chemo in ten to fourteen days. When they put the port in, they'll do a needle biopsy to determine if it's lung cancer or metastasized esophageal cancer. We'll get an MRI done in Hagerstown.

Today, we're navigating together, making plans on next steps. Whole new territory. And it still feels very unreal. I may be in shock.

John and I talked. He'll contact me, if possible, after he dies. The "plan" for now is he'll have Alice (our cat) knock something over or around on my desk. Amazing we had this conversation!

* * *

Today has been a mixed day: tears; talking about what John wants to get done before he starts chemo; Anne bringing over chicken soup for lunch; me researching some stuff for John; beginning weaving a new rug; ripping apart some curtains I got at Goodwill (very satisfying), prepping them for cutting into weaving rags; and many moments of life feeling normal. I'm hoping I sleep well tonight. I need it.

John is doing well. He's focused on getting some legal and financial stuff in order, as well as "eating" as much as he can. I so love that man.

Monday, February 18, 2019

Yesterday we both woke up angry. It was good. We got some stuff done.

John drafted a couple of letters: one to his gastro doc to see if there is any possibility of putting in a stent so he can eat more than 600-800 calories a day so he's in better physical shape to handle the chemo; and one to his chemo doc clarifying why he's so concerned about nutrition. I'll be reviewing them today for typos, etc. and John will send thru the cancer center portal AND overnight physical mail.

I was angry because I realized we'd been subjected to urban privilege, for lack of a better term. The medical oncologist had us pegged for country hicks. She didn't believe John had been a lawyer, then said "you're serious, aren't you" accompanied by a small giggle. I have it recorded. Not going to do anything with it for now because I don't want to muddy the waters. I get that telling someone you don't know that it looks like they have Stage 4 cancer and the prospects don't look good is difficult... but still, she could have done much better than that. Just sayin'.

In other news, I ripped out more seams on those curtains, washed and dried them. Now they are ready for cutting, when I'm ready.

I go up and down. I'm sooooooo very grateful for the antidepressant I'm on. It's making a huge difference in how well I'm handling all this.

* * *

On the getting things lined up side of things, instead of overnighting the letters, I faxed 'em.

Dr. Jafra (medical oncologist) called needing some info and it was a good exchange. She's working on getting approvals for the lung biopsy at the same time they put in the port. I now have her cell #. Win!!!!!

And – Dr. Morse, the gastro surgeon, called. John is scheduled for an endoscopy to put in a stent on Thursday at 11:30. We need to be there by 10:30. There will be two doctors working on him, one of them the one I saw 4 years ago who fixed my duodenal ulcer.

And – I've got someone lined up to plow the driveway and clean off my car so we can leave around 7:30.

And – I got the first 2 of 4 books I ordered on being a cancer patient caretaker.

All in all, a good day.

My transforaminal injection is scheduled for Wednesday, but I'm not sure I'll be able to make it cuz we're supposed to get 8-10 inches of snow with some sleet and freezing rain thrown in.

Monday, February 18, 2019

John to his group:

> *Hi everybody! Had a good day yesterday – felt very strong in spirit and got some things done. Working this week to get thru the list of must-dos, legal stuff, financial planning and making good progress. Received and accepted an offer of healing work from a group very experienced practitioners. I am feeling the support of my family and friends – thank you all!*

Tuesday, February 19, 2019

Today has been a good day and a hard day.

John asked that I set up an appointment with a financial advisor I know and am good friends with. She came up this morning to help John. The results were all we both had hoped for. And it was hard.

This afternoon, I went with John to his appointment with his attorney so he could sign a power of attorney and a medical power of attorney. I know it had to be done, and I'm crying that it had to be done. I hope I don't need to use them.

This not knowing… I don't have words to describe how hard it is.

And then there's this snow/ice storm coming in, starting late tonight and lasting 'til late tomorrow night.

John has an appointment for an endoscopy to put in a stent at the bottom of his esophagus so he can get more food into his body. It's for Thursday in Baltimore. I can drive in snow. I'm crap driving in snow and ice. His friend, Beau, is going to drive him. Beau's driving makes me car-sick. I feel relieved and guilty that I'll probably stay home Thursday, unless John really, really wants me there.

When I called this morning about the transforaminal injection for my sciatic nerve root inflammation, a wonderful thing happened. They totally got why I needed to cancel and they had an appointment opening next Monday! Yes!!!!!

John and I have had some good conversations today, sometimes a little tearful (on my part) and sometimes not. We both talked about how hard it was to be doing things to take care of the possibilities that he might be incapacitated or might die.

I realized I hadn't done any weaving yesterday and, even though it was almost midnight, I went and wove for 15-20 minutes. That helped settle me, too.

Tuesday, February 19, 2019

John to his group:

> *Some good news! I had written to my doctors in Balt asking to have an esophageal stent put in place so I could get more nutrition. I spend a huge amount of energy writing the letters, faxed them in monday about 11:00 am and got a call around 2 that I was scheduled for surgery next thurs Feb 21. A mighty coincidence. This is huge for me because my food intake is very limited and if successful, will give me more strength for the next part of this journey. Thanks to all for your support and help. Of course, there is the small matter of a foot of snow here tomorrow, but I have a real demolition derby driver lined up to drive me, we're going to take my old dented car and git 'er done getting to Baltimore on thurs!*

Thursday, February 21, 2019

John had the stent put in today. Dr. Morse said it went in easily and there were no complications. John is verrrrrrrry tired. He's in a little pain so he's staying on top of taking his (liquid) Percocet and Tylenol. The stent is one that expands and it will do so over the next 3-4 days. He's on a liquid diet until sometime tomorrow and then a little puréed food if his tummy can handle it. John is thrilled that he was able to drink water in more than little sips.

I had huge regrets that I didn't go today. I learned. From now on, I'm with John.

I also ended up having one of those times of deep, deep sobbing and crying. I needed that.

Tonight, it's beginning to sink in that I have a new full time "job."

Friday, February 22, 2019

John to his group:

Went down to Baltimore yesterday and they were able to install a stent so I can actually drink fluids more easily and will be able to eat soft foods soon! Hooray! Feel like a bunch of plumbers were playing in my throat but have meds to take care of that. I am looking at each step in treatment as a milestone, and this was a big one for improving the quality of my daily life. Love and thanks to all!

Pain is better today so I hope I won't be so zombified by the pain meds. Today we start to se if we can load some calories to get the motor turning over at more than a bare idle. :) A wild a crazy morning with some applesauce, a bottle of ensure, and a diet coke. Fluid is the bomb when you haven't been able to drink for a while. All my doctors are great and we are now planning for getting the chemo rolling next week. Not looking forward so much to that, but it's the next thing on the list to do.

> *I have a large portion of the kitchen counter covered with protein shake mixes, etc., and am taking other dietary supplements as well. Hard-boiled egg smoothies with chicken broth... .Will meet with a nutritionist next week in Balt. I'm lactose intolerant so I hadn't done any Ensure, but my wife found one that didn't have milk in it. Hopefully I will be able to move away from the stuff that has so much sugar and corn syrup in it. I was just grabbing calories wherever I could.*

Saturday, February 22, 2019

I'd ordered it Monday and it came yesterday. Today, I updated it. "It" being an 8½ inch by 11 inch appointment calendar. I was beginning to get confused trying to keep track of my appointments and John's appointments in two different calendars. The last thing I need is to double book one of us. Now that won't happen. I miss my little, purse size calendar and... it's OK.

Sunday, February 24, 2019

I'm doing way better than I was on Thursday. All of your comments have really helped. This whole experience is feeling seriouser and seriouser, unrealer and unrealer, and soooo unknown. I'm realizing that, yes I need to ask for help and... only I can deal with how I'm thinking/responding from inside. I'll ask for help with that too, and it's still an inside job. I'm still not sure what to ask for help with, beyond meals here and there for me. John's meals, when he gets beyond puréed in a day or so, have some restrictions. I'm hoping to get more info from a dietitian while John is getting his port placed.

I maybe overdid it a bit on Friday to make myself feel better, getting "things" done/arranged/etc. I'm noticing that I've got myself all wound up. Went to bed last night and couldn't get to sleep... for hours. Today, I'm being more conscious about taking Bach Flower Essence to calm me down. Tonight I'll have a cup of Kava tea before going to bed.

Part of it has been that I'm needing to do more. John is taking his pain meds (as he should) to help the healing where the stent was put in. He's sleeping a lot and when he's up, ummm, his brain isn't quite on target. It's almost like he's a different person. Definitely different from the John I've known these past 8+ years. It's partly the meds, and partly him letting go of being the tough guy and being vulnerable. Today, he took me up on my offer to do his laundry (he's always done his own, always!)

He shared, yesterday I think, that before he got the stent, he wasn't sure he'd make it through the winter. I had no idea he was thinking/feeling that. He said he thought it was unconscious because he didn't become aware of it himself until AFTER the stent was in place. As I watch how hard that treatment/surgery has hit him, I'm even more concerned about the chemo. I hope he gets a kind that doesn't waste the whole body, cuz I'm not sure he has the resources for that... and I remind myself that the human body can be incredibly resilient in situations one wouldn't think it could be.

The lung biopsy has been cancelled because the surgeon who would be doing it felt there was too high a possibility that, because of its position and how small the spot/tumor is, the procedure might collapse John's lung. Turns out that spot has grown from about 4 mm to about 7 mm (a little less than 1/4 inch to a little more than 1/4 inch) in 2 months. Not very big, but growing.

We'll be going down sometime next week for John to get the port, then home a few days so it can settle, then back for chemo. The chemo will be a mix of three drugs, two delivered in the infusion suite at the hospital, one from a bag over 24 hours, so we'll stay at Hope Lodge or somewhere else close that night. Dr. Jafra couldn't tell me the names of the chemo because HIPAA. I faxed my Medical Power of Attorney and a signed HIPAA Info release form today, so that doesn't happen again.

I've been reading two books in particular that have been helpful but... I Need. To. Take. A. Break from them!

They have wonderful info. *Things I Wish I'd Known* by Deborah J. Cornwall has soooo much info that other cancer caregivers offered the author for her book. *A Hospice Chaplain's Field Guide to Caregiving* by E.M. Hager is more spiritually oriented, without being at all preachy!

I'm getting huge hints that this experience is going to be a huge roller coaster for John and for me.

I'm working on a new short story about cancer. We'll see how that goes. It feels like a way to process some of this.

Sunday, February 24, 2019

John is still having pain from the placement of the stent in his esophagus to his stomach. It's about a 3, down from a 6, which is good. However, he has a sharp pain in the middle of his back that wasn't there before the stent placement and has been there ever since.

Monday, February 25, 2019

Yay! It's only been four days since John got the stent and today he ate a half can of Progresso Chunky Soup! He reports that his stomach feels unsure about it, but it's handling it.

John's back still hurts. Enough that it's interfering with his sleep. He's taking 4 – 6 doses of 5 ml Percocet a day now, along with ibuprofen and acetaminophen. He hasn't needed nausea meds though!

Tuesday, February 26, 2019

Today was a good day.

Yesterday, I finally got my injection in my lower back. It's already helping. And I've got the next one scheduled. Hopefully I won't need it, but if I do, it's already set up.

Today I saw Margi, my therapist, for the first time in 2 weeks. I have hope back. And breathing. She introduced me to Stillpoint, a small building on her property that is sacred and beautiful. I walked in and could feel the stillness immediately. Everything in me relaxed.

The other thing I'm finally getting is that this whole thing is one huge learning experience, I have zero control over what's going to happen, and I will make mistakes. I'll do the best I can with what I know in the moment and go on from there. And… knowing me, I'll get to re-realize this innumerable times.

Joyce brought me dinner tonight: roast chicken with potatoes, carrots, and cauliflower. It was sooooo good. A real meal.

Which brings me to: asking for help. I don't know what I'll need help with. If you have something you'd like to do, please ask me if I'd like _____. I can then answer yes or no. If you ask "what can I do" I mostly can't think of anything in the moment because there is already so much I'm now taking care of and I've no idea what's coming. I can say that if you like to cook, I could use help with that for me, especially if it can be frozen. I suck at cooking for myself. John's diet now has a bunch of restrictions and there will probably be more after I, hopefully, get to talk to a dietician when we're in Baltimore next week.

John had a rougher day. We now have a date for getting his port inserted (next Monday), with chemo starting probably on Thursday next week. It has moved from theoretical to real for him. He's scared. I don't blame him, not one bit! I would be too if it was me. His body is still adjusting to the stent so he's in pain. Better than it was… and still there. Still needing the Percocet.

Knowing all of you are here is huge for me. I don't feel alone as we continue this journey into a very unpredictable future. Thank you for being my kith and kin.

Wednesday, February 27, 2019

John's chemo is scheduled for next Thursday, March 7. We'll need to go down Wednesday evening because he needs to be there at 8:15 for labs (we'll find out what that means), with 4 hours of chemo starting at 9:10. Then they'll attach a bag of another chemo that will go for 24 hours. We'll return to the cancer center Friday morning for them to remove it, then we come home.

The cancer center staff are telling us everyone reacts differently to chemo and there's no way to tell ahead of time. John's reaction might be the same day or delayed for several (or more) days. I've noticed that I'm getting bits of information before I need them. Often enough that it's more than coincidence.

Gulp. I think I'm in shock. It's now really, really real.

Looking Back

Setting up my *Kith and Kin* group and John setting up his *Planning for John's 70th Birthday Party* group made all the difference for both of us. I had a safe place to share what I was experiencing and John had a group of his friends and healers to whom he could go for help.

Two things stand out for me about this time.

First – Months later, Beau told me that when John was in recovery after the stent surgery, he was terrified. He asked Beau to hold his hand, which Beau did. I never let John go anywhere without me again. Whatever the time or the weather, I drove him or rode with him if Beau was driving. It also brought John and Beau closer and that was a blessing for John. As things progressed, Beau was there for John as a close friend.

Second – The hints I was getting about things were such a blessing. There were spirits around that were making sure I knew what I needed to know when I needed to know it. While I'm not generally aware of that sort of thing, living with the strong possibility of John's death broke me open to having that kind of extra awareness.

PART IV:
CHEMO

Friday, February 28, 2019

I've had a rough couple days. I messed up taking my meds and my anti-depressant Was. Not. Happy, and therefore I wasn't. It's evened out now. Another lesson learned.

AND… for 2 days in a row now, John has eaten real food for breakfast (2 scrambled eggs with deviled ham in them) and for dinner Stouffer's chicken, veggies, & rice, which is comfort food for him and he can "cook" it himself! He also ate half a banana today. I'm not sure what else he ate, and that's ok. His stent is still a little tender, but he chews small bites slowly and it goes into his stomach, instead of getting caught and coming back up and out. His back pain is much less, so he's getting about 8 hours of sleep at night. These are both HUGE improvements!

Tomorrow, we go to Hagerstown (1 hour away) for John's thoracic MRI to see what's going on with his T12 vertebrae. It's supposed to snow tonight, but should be fine by the time we leave at noon.

I'm keeping an eye on the forecasts for Sunday/Monday. We need to be in Baltimore (2 hours away) by 9:30 so they can put his port in. If it looks like it seriously wants to snow, we'll go down Sunday and spend the night.

He has to be in Baltimore again on Thursday by 8:15, so I've already made reservations for us for Wednesday and Thursday, since he'll have to go back to the infusion center Thursday to have the 24 hour chemo bag removed. Then we'll repeat this every 2 weeks. Not sure for how long. I'm really glad it looks like winter and snow threats are fading away!

Please keep us in your prayers, meditations, thoughts, and rituals that John's chemo works without making him feel awful and that I can be kind to myself so I can be kind to him.

Friday, March 1, 2019

John to his group:

> Hi everybody, making progress slow but sure. Had an MRI today which I thought would just be an annoying event, but turned into a little more. The way they had me on the table really aggravated my back pain – which started after my last procedure – could barely hold it through the MRI. But it is done. The stent is settling in, and I can eat more, but it is still kind of hit or miss between appetite and pain from the procedure. Overall better though.
>
> Finished up all the estate planning whirlwind except need to sign a few more documents. Thinking part is done. Next week will be a double Baltimore week. Chemo port installed on Monday, Chemo starts on thursday.
>
> Looking forward to spring.

Saturday, March 2, 2019

Yesterday was a hard day for John. He had an MRI to check out the spot on his T12 vertebrae. Having to lie still soooo long in an uncomfortable position on a hard surface and all the banging, his back really hurt and his tinnitus kicked up major in both ears by the time they freed him from The Machine. He's doing lots better today.

We head to Baltimore early Monday morning so he can get his port. His friend, Beau, is going to drive us cuz it's supposed to snow 5+ inches Sunday afternoon/night and Beau knows how to drive in that in traffic. John said it makes it easier for him cuz he won't worry about me getting tired. Yay Beau!

AND… Sally is bringing me dinner on Tuesday; and Jenn has treated me to Purple Carrot, which will deliver the ready to use ingredients for 3 meals on March 13! Thank you, thank you, thank you to you both!

Posting here helps me stay clear on what's going on, with myself and with John.

* * *

This reality of John's cancer is settling in in my awareness and consciousness.

There is grief. There is now also acceptance. This will kill him and it will do so in 6 – 12 months. I don't get the feeling it will even be that long.

The stent he had put in February 21 so he can eat has really taken it out of him. There's a lot more pain involved. His mid-back has hurt fairly constantly since then. Percocet kinda keeps it under control. I've got a sinking feeling that that pain isn't a "left over" from the surgery. I think it's cancer in his T12 vertebrae.

John will never in this life and this body be cured of the cancer. It is killing him. The pain and the meds are changing him, as they must.

Dr. Grant said today my main job is to be John's advocate and record keeper. Anything else I can do is limited (my awareness).

Because of my own back (I had a microdiscectomy in July, 2018 and it's all still healing) there is little I can do to help him physically if he gets too weak or falls.

I can make sure he takes any meds on time.

It's almost 4 in the morning. I couldn't sleep, so I got up.

This shit is real. John is going to die of this sometime this year.

I'm scared the chemo is going to kill him. He's already so weak and debilitated because he hasn't been able to eat more than 600 – 800 calories a day for several months. He has so little physical resilience.

I don't even have tears right now. I know I will, but right now? None. My stomach is upset. A form of shock?

It feels like this reality is settling in. The John I knew well will not be returning in this lifetime.

The medical oncologist wanted to get started on the chemo ASAP, within 2 weeks of our first visit on February 15. It will be 3 weeks. But if John hadn't gotten the stent... and I wonder if the stent has released more cancer cells in his body. John said he didn't think he'd see spring and hadn't realized that until after the stent was placed.

He's still not eating that much.

I just need to get all this out so I can put a good face on it when John's awake.

And – I spend a lot of time alone these days. He's sleeping a lot.

He's expended a lot of energy to make sure his legal and financial affairs are in order and to make sure I'll be taken care of going forward.

I keep reminding myself of two things:

- the vision I had about 15 years ago of myself in a long flowing blue dress, short white hair, holding a bright flower while standing in a field of blooming zinnias in so many colors.
- a feeling/sense I had shortly after I moved in with John in April of 2011 that there would be challenging physical illnesses happening in this house and deciding that I'd take that risk because of the love between John and me.

Monday, March 4, 2019

John has his port. It's a little tender right now and he understands why they don't start chemo right away. He was awake while they put it in and talked with the doctor while it was happening. They had a drape over his head so he couldn't see what was happening. He said it felt strange, as they got the tubing into his vein.

We didn't get as much snow as predicted (thank you) but it was enough to make the back roads a bit slushy and slick. Beau got us there in plenty of time.

I'm really tired tonight. Not sure why and… I am. So I'll be going to bed by 10, which is early for me.

Wednesday we go back down so John can start chemo Thursday.

Tomorrow we go see the lawyer so John can finalize his will and trust. I see Margi at 2. And I'll figure out what we'll be taking to Baltimore: mini room humidifier, charging cords, various pillows and fleece blankets, a walker (on the principle "if we have it we won't need it"), and…? I'll definitely be using one of those hotel cart thingies.

In an odd way, these past two days have felt kind of normal, almost like before all this came to light. I'm appreciating it while it's here.

As soon as I post this, I'm going to tie a few more knots on the edge of a rug. I'll remember, hopefully tomorrow, to take a picture of the rugs I've taken off the loom.

It feels like I'm trying to establish a new normal. And we're both hoping the chemo goes well without bad side effects.

Monday, March 4, 2019

John to his group:

Another trip to Balt today to get a chemo port installed. Success! But it's pretty weird to have people numb up your neck and chest and then start saying things like "you may feel some pain" while they are doing who knows what to your neck. Some pain is correct, esp. when they are squishing everything arounds. But the deed is done thanks to my friend who drove us and my dear wife, who makes sure we go to the right building and is doing so much for me to make this easier.

Wednesday, March 6, 2019

John to his group:

> *Back to Balt today to be there bright and early for chemo tommorow at 8 am. I'm starting to feel like a 7th grade science project with all the extra parts they keep adding on me. Pain from getting port is setting down, not something I hope to repeat again soon.*

Wednesday, March 6, 2019

We got to Baltimore in good time and we're settled into our room. Nervous, scared? Yes. And John is feeling stronger physically, and clear and held spiritually.

I'm also in a space of calm.

Caryn came to our hotel room to do a ritual/healing for John. She brought *The Journey Into Spirit* by Kristoffer Hughes. As I fanned through the pages, my eyes landed on the paragraph at the end of a chapter.

"Nobody should have to die alone, isolated in their own fear. Consider the importance of training in soul midwifery or another death and dying-related program that serves your community. What can you do in service to those who will die?" (p129)

I've been considering this for several years. This isn't the time, that will be later.

As Caryn was doing the Reiki attunement with Bridget's fire, I held space, calling in St. Catherine of Sienna. I remembered, as I haven't in quite a while, a dream I had years ago that had the phrase "the healing hands of St. Catherine," with a shaft of green light coming down from the sky and St. Catherine walking through rubble where there were nobles who were injured, ill, or dying. It's time to revisit that.

Caryn shared a phrase she used during her two bouts with cancer: "I'm alive today and I'll be alive tomorrow."

March 7, 2019

Shortly, we're leaving to start this chemo process for real, instead of thinking about it. I'll keep you updated.

* * *

We've met a LOT of people so far. John's actual infusion started about an hour ago. He's high on steroids and feeling relief treatment has started. I'm still pretty much in my state of calm.

There's a lot to absorb, information wise. I'm just taking it moment by moment.

* * *

We got back to the hotel around 4 and we both took naps. John's loaded up with steroids, so he's not feeling much from the chemo yet. They said it would be 4-5 days. He's happily at his laptop, catching up on Brexit news and other stuff. He's had dinner. It's soooo wonderful to see him eating. He's gained 5 pounds since he got his stent!

Me? I'm pooped. Didn't sleep well last night or the night before. Hopefully, now that it's underway, I'll get sleep tonight.

Thursday, March 7, 2019

John to his group:

1st chemo session done! 8 am to 3 30 at the hospital. long day. met with all kinds of doctors nurses social workers, etc. Lots of info. Still have a 24 hr bottle of potion #99 hooked up which will be removed tomorrow, then home fri or sat depending on when hosp stuff gets finished. Hosp staff ws great.

Friday, March 8, 2019

John is now free of the 24 hour chemo bottle. He's reveling in not having to be conscious of it when he's taking a nap or just moving around. Still no side-effects, for which we're both grateful. They told us, again, that it will probably be 5-6 days before they show up.

We're spending tonight in Baltimore. His chemo bottle wasn't ready (i.e. empty) for removal until around 4 this afternoon. We'd suspected that would be the timing and opted to drive home in the morning with NO rush hour.

John wants spaghetti and meatballs for dinner. This is sooooo do-able.

I'm feeling a little more rested. I took a caretaker stress test earlier today on one of the cancer websites. Ummmm... I'm stressed. I'll take it again when I get home to see what the questions are, how I answer them, and ask for help from there.

We're both ready to be HOME!!

Update: welp... spaghetti and meatballs was a hit. He enjoyed every bite. John assures me that he has a good sense of what his body can handle. He ate a little too much, too fast (I totally understand) plus he had 2 bites of garlic bread. Bread is on the Do Not Eat List for his stent. I could hear his body talking to him.

My choice was either be an I-told-you-so nag or exit the room. It feels waaaaay healthier (and safer for his feelings) than me trying to suppress the grin that would have gone with the I-told-you-so. The fact he didn't come with me for the post-dinner cig speaks volumes. It doesn't feel serious, just kinda funny, like a kid testing the limits.

Saturday, March 9, 2019

This is a bit of this/bit of that post.

We got home about noon today. Sooooo glad we didn't try it last night.

Now that we're home, I've discovered I'm exhausted. Not really a surprise when I think about it.

John's taken several naps and he's taking his nausea meds cuz… nausea. I hope it doesn't get too bad, but it will be what it will be.

There will be three more chemo sessions, one every two weeks, and then a scan to see how the tumors are doing. They'll also take blood work before we get there to make sure his liver and kidneys are in good shape to handle the chemo.

Everything he drinks now has to be hot or at room temp. Nothing cold because the chemo meds may very well make him very sensitive to cold and can make his throat feel like it's closing, even though it isn't. If it happens, it will last about three days, give or take. By the second week after the chemo, he should be less sensitive.

We need to keep track of his body temperature, his sleep patterns and a bunch of other stuff. I knew chemo was serious stuff, but I had no idea how many body systems it can mess with!

The hotel had a decent sized mini fridge that was nice and cold. Therefore: we have leftovers! I'm happy I don't have to think about what I'll be eating for the next few days.

What is it about us humans? Like John, I had to test my own limits. I know full well that if I'm not careful about how much sugar I eat I get migraines. I wanted something sweet while we were in Baltimore. Predictably, I had a migraine 2 nights running, and needed my migraine med both nights. Sigh. I'm being very, very, very good now that I'm home.

Tomorrow I get to see my acupuncturist. I need it!

Ok. I think that's it

Oh, nope. Thank you all for being here. It makes such a difference to know I'm so lovingly supported.

Sunday, March 10, 2019

John to his group:

> *Back home at last. Whew! Feeling decent today, no immediate big reaction to chemo, except some nausea, but able to eat ok. It is quite an experience to be hooked up to all those bags of jungle juice in the hospital, and then to have one hanging around your neck for 24 hrs.*
>
> *Big thanks to my friend Caryn who came by wed eve and did a Brighid healing ceremony on me at the hotel before the chemo. To all my "witch doctor" friends, keep rattlin' the drums, it's working. To all my family and friends here, many thanks — you are keeping my spirit strong!*

Sunday, March 10, 2019

Local folks — do any of you have a coffee table that needs a new home? I have my old oval cherry one, which is pretty, but oval takes up too much room in our tiny living room and John will be using the living room more as we journey further down this path. He'll need a place for his water, his diet coke, books, etc.

I'd be happy to do a swap, if that works.

Thank you all for the food you've dropped by. It's pretty much for me right now since John is sticking to his diet of frozen food or me scrambling eggs.

Tuesday, March 14, 2018

John has had nausea the past couple of days that his nausea prescriptions aren't touching. He's not eating much and he's not sleeping much. He's a little better in the morning, then progressively worse as the day goes on. He stays lying down a lot because the nausea is less when he is.

Maybe TMI here and… he had some nausea suppositories from when he got the stent. He used the last one last night and had less nausea and slept better. I'm checking with Dr. Jafra today to see if we can get another prescription for them.

Saturday, March 16, 2019

John to his group:

Feeling the spring energy now, and think I'm through the worst of the chemo for now. Nasty stuff. We got our driveway fixed so it's not mud city and they may be able to help with some other stuff.

My gratitude is increasing every day for the opportunity to get good treatment for this. It wasn't until the weather finally started to break that I believed I was going to make it through the winter. Winter was 99% crazy because I was sick and couldn't eat. Primordial fear of starvation is a pretty weird thing to experience. Not being able to eat for so long really turns you inside emotionally and physically.

Blessings to all my friends and family who are providing such wonderful support. And of course, to my wife for her tireless organization and advocacy navigating my treatment And my cat Alice who spends countless hours lying next to me in bed purring and batting me on the nose if she thinks I look funny.

Saturday, March 16, 2019

A couple of things.

John posted in his Facebook group today. I'm so glad he took my suggestion seriously and set up his own group. It's a funny mix for me, reading his posts. I learn things he hasn't shared with me (his fear he wouldn't survive through the winter) and I see how he's making things sound a little better than they are (giving the impression that he's finally able to eat, without even saying that).

The chemo is starting to seriously kick John's butt, especially the nausea, which means he can't eat, which means he's hungry, which makes his esophagus/stent kinda hurt, and it's a cycle that the usual nausea meds weren't quite handling. I called Dr. Jafra yesterday and she said to call/see Dr. Grant (our GP). I now understand why. She was recommending a steroid and Xanax. The Xanax I had to carry a paper script to the pharmacy to fill, can't be called/faxed in. Because John gave me his Medical Power of Attorney, I can pick it up, instead of him having to. We didn't think I'd need it so soon. John slept MUCH better last night and he was able to eat a light dinner and then breakfast this morning.

I'm in a philosophical place, for lack of a better description. Things are what they are. Nothing much I can do but be with what's up. I'm also becoming more aware of a kind of cycle re: the feelings I'm experiencing in a day and over the course of a week (give or take).

And... on Wednesday, a Purple Carrot delivery arrived at my door (big Thank You to Jenn!) Pretty amazing packaging. So's the food. Last night, I made the Tempeh Vegetable Korma. I love Korma! There's lots of the sauce left over, so I can use it on other meals.

Today, it will be Crispy Quinoa Cakes. (I just noticed it looks like I'm going in the order they were packed in the box, lol). I'm amazed at how filling this plant based food is!

Monday, March 18, 2019

I've sent a request to Dr. Jafra to move our check-in time at the infusion center from 11 to 10 on Friday, since we're getting John's kidney/liver blood work done locally this week and sent over to them.

Tuesday, March 19, 2019

I've been thinking about the "philosophical place" I've been in. Talking to Margi about it, she suggested it might be a feeling of peace. That fits much better. Peace as in: there's nothing I can do to change or control what's happening for John. It is what it is, regardless of how I feel about it. Fighting that doesn't work. Peace does. It leaves me with more energy to do the small things I can do: scrambling him some eggs, fetching something for him from somewhere else in the house, washing his clothes, picking up meds, calling doctors, etc.

I'll hold on to the peace, gently. I've learned over the years that holding on fiercely doesn't work as well. But oh how I wish things were different!

We leave on Thursday for Baltimore and round 2 of chemo. John's energy is much diminished. He sleeps/naps probably 18 hours out of every day. He's exhausted. Mornings are good. As the day progresses, I can see him going deeply inward. I know he's tired.

Dr. Jafra approved starting chemo at 10 instead of 11. It will be 4 hours on Friday, then the 24 hour bottle, which will be removed on Saturday. We'll stay Saturday night. I figure he'll be pretty tired out. And… I'll feel better knowing that, if something goes sideways with how he responds to the chemo, we're already in Baltimore.

Wednesday, March 20, 2019

John to his group:

Many thanks to all. Last couple of days were pretty challenging. Chemo kicks you ass in 16 different ways. Feeling a bit better today. Back to Balt tomorrow to get ready for Chemo2 on Friday.

Wednesday, March 20, 2019

I had a meltdown this morning. I suspected it was coming because I seriously wanted to flip a driver off when I was driving John to Hagerstown, which is an hour from home. We had to go there for his blood draw to see if his liver, kidneys, and white blood count are good enough for chemo round 2. Going to the satellite office (which is only 20 minutes away) hadn't worked last time, so I didn't want to risk that again.

Flipping off drivers is *not* one of my "things". Then, when we got home and John was sleeping, I discovered I'd forgotten I'd washed some of John's clothes a few days ago and they were still in the washer, musty smelling. And two light bulbs burned out in the kitchen. Normally, no big deal. Today, they tipped me further over the edge. I broke down in tears of anger and grief, wailing "it's just not fair!" That John has terminal cancer, that our future together is nothing like we envisioned, that he's so weak and feels so crappy, that I'm losing things, and I got a package today that I thought I'd cancelled.

I grabbed my dammit doll and whacked away at the door frame between the kitchen and the office. There were whacks for the unfairness of it all; whacks for the grief of John becoming less and less "here" as he deals with his own grief and pain; whacks for John's suffering and how little I can do. It's just hard. I had to let it out. Had to. I've learned the hard way that if I don't, ignored feelings will come back at me later harder and fiercer. I feel a bit more grounded, but the grief is still there. I suspect it will be for quite a while.

And yes, that peace is still under all this, but right now it's not front and center. It's hard staying positive. I know this cancer is killing him, sooner rather than later. It's heart wrenching seeing how awful the chemo is making him feel, on top of him already being exhausted because he can't eat enough. And chemo brain. It's robbing him of his wit, his mental quickness, his ability to think or even remember things. Being here doesn't feel like enough, but I hear from so many that it's the most important thing.

I'm doing my best to stay positive when I'm around him because it's one of the things I can do.

It's a good thing I'm seeing my acupuncturist this afternoon. It's also a good thing I saw Margi yesterday and have a new breathing tool (big sigh, making noise on the outbreath).

I'm so glad I have my secret Facebook support group. You hear my pain, acknowledge it, and I "talk" about the things that I won't talk about with John. I don't think he needs to know all my ins and outs dealing with this. He's got enough. And he loves me so much that he'd try to do something to help.

My friend, Sally, asked me to come over and take a walk with her. I'll take her up on that when the weather is nicer. My back is still healing and uneven ground makes it worse.

She made me some acorn squash and meatloaf. They're delicious! I'm having seconds tonight and freezing the rest.

I just saw John's post to his own Facebook group. I'm crying.

Thursday, March 21, 2019

John to his group:
> *Woke up this morning with NO nausea and NO pain for the first time in weeks. What a blessing!*

Thursday, March 21, 2019

We're here. Driving was intense with rain, fog, and the water that cars and trucks generously splashed up. Coming down the night before is working well for us.

I'm in focused mode. And taking time to breathe and not think too much about anything except right now.

Friday, March 22, 2019

John to his group:

> *Achievement Earned !*
> *Chemo LvL 2 Badge awarded!*
> *Not too bad today, they took one of the nasty potions out of the rotation for this round. should help with nausea. was at the hospital from 10-4 , all the staff was great.*

Sunday, March 24, 2019

We're back home, tired but doing well.

We stayed at a different hotel this time and got a suite with 2 queens and a separate living area with a microwave and fridge. It wasn't a whole lot more than the room we had two weeks ago and... it was absolutely worth it. John rarely sleeps through the night. This arrangement let him get up when he needed to without worrying about disturbing me.

The staff there is amazing: friendly, helpful, cheerful.

John ended up having an hour long conversation with a security guard. The man's ex and his mother both have cancer. John was able to share what he's learned, what he knows, who he is. He ended up getting a hug from the man. It was an affirming and powerful interaction for John.

On the medical side of things, John's liver numbers were too high so Dr. Jafra only gave him 2 of the chemo drugs, instead of 3. His blood pressure was also really low, so, on doctor's orders, he's stopped taking his blood pressure med. We're hoping his nausea won't be as bad this time around. We'll find out.

Yesterday, I'd had enough. Frustrated, feeling overwhelmed, tired. I told John he IS going to go into remission for a loooong time cuz I'm not going thru all this for nothing. He laughed and agreed. He then went on to talk about what he wants to get done in the next 6 or so months, since, in our meeting with her on February 15, Dr. Jafra gave him 6-12 months, with a VERY tentative "maybe more" tacked on to the end of her prognosis. Somehow, me making that statement is allowing me to be more present and at peace with where we are right now. I realized I had been living in a lot of fear and it was creating way too much self-inflicted stress. There is now room inside me for hope. Maybe John can be one of those who beats the odds. It doesn't feel like denial. It feels like opening up to possibilities. Besides which, with everything else I'm doing, it's just too tiring to project a future without him. Yes, it's likely, and… he's alive right now and for an unknown number of weeks and months. It's one day at a time right now, sometimes one hour or one minute. I'm learning (and experiencing) ever deeper levels of what not being in control really is. I'm grateful that John is a strong willed man, with a huge heart. It's allowing him to experience all of this with grace.

Today I ordered a shower bench, the kind where half of it is outside the tub, the other half inside. And a new shower head, with a long hose. John can't get in the shower or stand long enough to take one. They'll be here in a few days.

I'm really hoping this second round of chemo isn't as bad as the first. We'll find out.

Tuesday, March 26, 2019

John to his group:

Whoa, that was some "special" chemo I got last friday, flat on my ass sunday and mon with horrible nausea. Better today with more steroids and meds. First time on the internet in two days – it was making me dizzy.

Witch Doctor Version: Tyr and Gleipnir hold the wolf firm and wolfie is pissed, tearing out his own hair and beard. Brighid's yellow green fire slowly surrounds and consumes the wolf, and draws the residue into her furnace and then gone.

In prayer and meditiation this morning, received a visit from the spirits of my mother, her sister and brother. No communication, just a presence that they are around and will help. Major omen for me.

Thursday, March 28, 2019

John updated his group cover photo.

Our new home away from home in Baltimore – hotel has Zappa hanging in main lobby, and other 60s 70s stars in the rooms. We had Jerry Garcia in the bathroom.

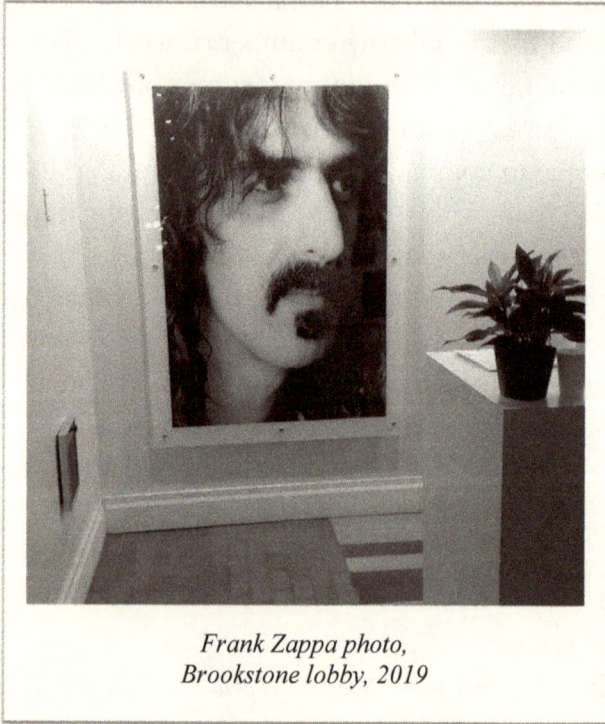

Frank Zappa photo,
Brookstone lobby, 2019

Saturday, March 30, 2019

It's been a week since John began his 2nd round of chemo. He's miserable. The nausea is back in force and his mouth and throat are covered in sores and it hurts to talk, drink, eat, swallow. Between nausea and the mouth/throat sores, he's back to eating maybe 800-1000 calories a day.

Dr. Jafra prescribed something called "Magic Mouthwash" – it has lidocaine in it. It helps, sort of. I understand more and more why people who've had chemo shake their heads, say they're sorry, and that there's no way to describe the experience.

The only thing I know to do is just be here for him. I get teary now and again. Mostly I keep myself busy doing things for him and doing things for me. Staying present remains the key. When I catch myself looking forward, I stop myself. It's easier.

At this point, I don't even see how he can go through another round starting next Friday. I remind myself that bodies are more resilient than we think. I'm just not sure how much resilience John has left. He's a strong man. He's determined to make this work. I sooooo hope it does.

Morning update: his mouth doesn't hurt as much, mucus is down, he got some good sleep, and he has a little more energy. YAY!!!!

Sunday, March 31, 2019

Soooo… it's been a verrrrrry lonnnnng day.

John's mouth (and its mucus production) got worse as the day progressed. Then late last night (like 1 in the morning) he mentioned that his feet were really swollen, with the right one feeling numb and hard to move his toes. Oh. I excused myself to get something for him, and had to push down tears of fear that peripheral neuropathy might be showing up.

I called the patient help line at UMMC and the doctor who called back strongly recommended we go to the ER. We left at 2 in the morning, driving to Hagerstown, about 50 minutes away. John was discharged a little after 2 this afternoon. I had moments of wondering if I'd done the right thing, taking him up there. I now know it was absolutely the right thing. The UMMC doctor said something that really struck me: that I'm not only an advocate for John with health care people, I'm an advocate for John with himself.

Turns out he has thrush, big time. The swelling in his feet is probably due to the lack of protein, cuz it hurts to eat and swallow.

The hospitalist gave him an antifungal to start working on getting the thrush under control, as well as a prescription. He also got IV fluid, as well as IV potassium (which was low again cuz he couldn't eat).

I go to RiteAid after we get home. They don't have the antifungal the hospitalist prescribed. No non-hospital pharmacies do. It "disappeared" 3-4 months ago. The pharmacist showed me what is being prescribed instead. I was in tears at that news. I ended up texting our GP (Dr. Grant). He got right back to me and said he'd call in a prescription.

I then took a short nap. I'd been up for something like 36 hours at that point. I got back to the pharmacy at 6:30. They closed at 6. Major tears because I was making John's pain last longer because I didn't get right down there. And what he's going through right now is major awful. He's got some questions he wants to ask Dr. Jafra this coming Friday.

I can't remember the last time I was awake for this long. I do remember that it takes more than one night to "recover."

I fessed up to John and apologized for causing him more suffering, crying as I told him. I couldn't help it. He asked me to come sit with him on the couch. He held me and said it was really ok. That what they gave him in the ER was already helping. And that he wasn't sure he could have done what I just did: the driving, dealing with ER staff, staying awake, being there for and with him. He's such a special man. I'm all weepy just writing this.

And I'm so tired. And I will be at Rite Aid when they open at 8 tomorrow morning.

Thank you for being here and for loving us both.

* * *

Update: John just told me he's going to tell his oncologist that he can't go through this again right now and that he'd like to revisit his treatment plan. I agree.

Sunday, March 31, 2019

John to his group:

What a week. Ended up spending 12 hours in an ER in Hagerstown last night. In a wheelchair. Will spare you all the gritty details, but last week's chemo resulted in a full blown thrush infection in my mouth with hundred of sores, feet swollen so big couldn't walk, etc. Got multiple IV infusions including anti-nausea meds, fluids, potassium supplements and who knows what else. Meds on order for thrush and should knock it out in a few days and then I will hopefully be able to eat again.

What a miserable ride this week has been. There is no way I can be physically ready to do the next chemo session, so will talk to my Dr about that.

* * *

Thanks to all for your love, prayers and support. Letting the Dr know there isn't going to be any chemo next week until I heal up.

Thursday, April 4, 2019

A quick update. First: John has decided NOT to go to Baltimore for his third round of chemo on Friday. I'm in total agreement and support. He needs time to build his body back up again. We faxed his test results and a letter to them on Monday, asking for a review of his treatment plan.

I'm beginning to feel human again, as in enough sleep and oh so many dreams! Feels like it may take another couple days to recover from the all-nighter. I'm not surprised, lol.

Friday, April 5, 2019

John to his group:

> *Things have finallyu settled down with my body and I'm doing better than last week. Next chemo session is postponed pending review of treatment paln. I was supposed to be there today sure glad I am not. whew.*

> *I got most of my hair cut off 2 weeks ago to prepare for when it started to come out, but it kept coming out and I ended feeling like a shaggy dog that was shedding all over my clothes, so went back to the barber.*

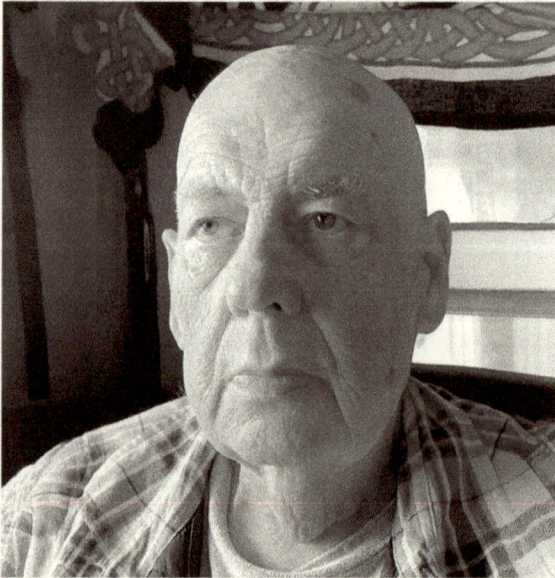

John, after the barber's visit, 2019

Tuesday, April 9, 2019

John to his group:

> *Enough already, body finally starting to get well, now I have cellulitis in my right leg. Started on oral antibiotics, may need to get intravenous antibiotics if it doesn't clear quickly. Some day, I will have a day without a doctor app't and nothing to do but sit in the sun.*
>
> *Went back to the doc this am and will stay on the oral antibiotics for now. Really don't want to play ER again this soon. Wonderful folks, but let them help someone else for a while.*

Tuesday, April 9, 2019

John has really bad cellulitis that's blistering. His feet and lower legs are really swollen. He's on oral antibiotics today and sees Dr. Grant tomorrow. If no improvement, he'll be going to the hospital for a few days for IV antibiotics. Dr. Grant is concerned sepsis could happen. God damn fucking chemo and it's fucking "side effects"! I don't think John realizes how serious it is. At this point, I'm not going to tell him.

Thursday, April 11, 2019

John to his group:

> *A little spring creeping in with the peach tree starting to blossom.*

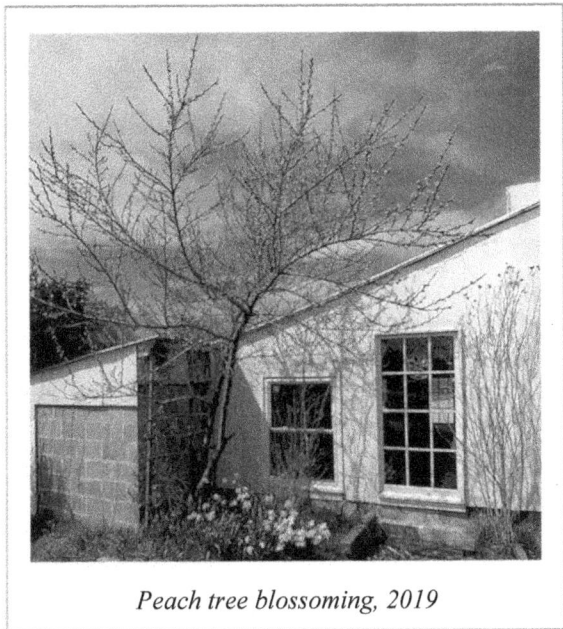

Peach tree blossoming, 2019

Saturday, April 13, 2019

John's dad, Ero (his partner), Mara (Ero's daughter), and David (Mara's boyfriend) came up for a visit today. It was good. John absolutely had to see his father. I think they both needed to see each other and confirm that they were both ok. John's father, btw, is 97.

Monday, April 15, 2019

John to his group:

Had a nice family visit with my dad on saturday. His partner's daughter drove them up and brough lots of goodies.

Back to the dr today on my legs – the short answer is going to be go to the ER and get IV antibiotics. I'm hoping I don't have to stay there, but at this point, whatever happens, happens. Other than my legs, feel pretty good today.

Monday, April 15, 2019

Things are kinda-sorta progressing. John's thrush is under control. However… he has cellulitis in his feet and lower legs. Oral antibiotics and shots are NOT taking care of it. He really, really doesn't want to go to the hospital, but it's looking more and more like the only thing that will work is IV antibiotics. Dr. Grant is strongly recommending he go. We'll see Dr. Grant tomorrow and, if there's no improvement, John's agreed he'll go.

We heard from his oncologist on Friday. No more chemo until everything is cleared up (thrush, cellulitis) and he's gained some weight. At that point, we'll be offered options, which may include chemo lite or no chemo. Radiation is not in the picture until/unless the chemo works.

Me? It took a good week to recover from the all-night marathon. I'm definitely NOT 20 (or 40) anymore!

I'm in a place of feeling pretty alone. It's a different kind of loneliness than I've ever felt before; a deep, inner loneliness. It doesn't matter whether I'm physically alone or not, it's always present. It's also making it difficult for me to ask for help, mostly because I've no idea what to ask for. I suspect part of that is decision fatigue.

Time is kinda weird. Some things seem ages ago and they were only days ago, other things seem like yesterday and they were who knows how long ago.

I continue to weave rugs. Sometime recently (it's that time thing) I found a treasure: a 1920's/30's era kitchen cabinet with glass doors. Habitat for Humanity ReStore in Winchester for the win! It cost me a whole $65. I love it!! It's now storing the used fabrics and clothing I'll be cutting into rags for rugs. Seeing all the colors and patterns is such a treat.

And I've woven three more rag rugs. It's soothing for me and John likes to hear the thump as I beat the weft.

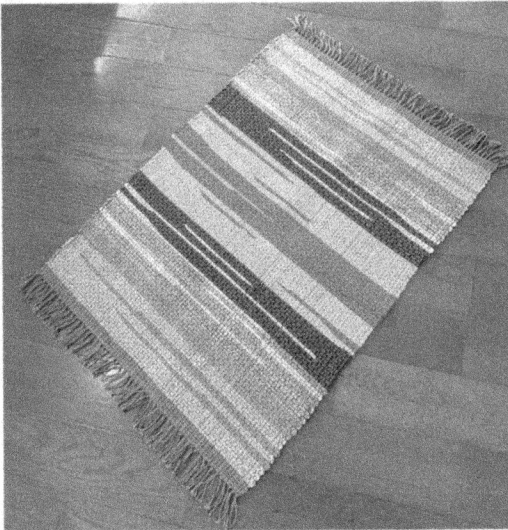

One of Elmdea's rag rugs:
Earth, Sea, and Sky, 2019

Looking Back

Chemo – it's such wicked stuff. I know there weren't really any other options, but John's quality of life declined so quickly, it didn't feel right then and it still doesn't feel right. But it was the only option available to him other than doing nothing. John wanted to do everything he could to live as long as he could. For starters, he wanted to see his grandbabies grow up.

I now have a better understanding of my feelings of deep aloneness. There wasn't anyone I could talk to who'd been through a similar experience. Later, in a hospice grief group, everyone knew. It would have been immeasurably worse without my *Kith & Kin* group.

PART V:
CHANGING ONCOLOGISTS

Tuesday, April 16, 2019

BIG sigh of relief! John is now safely ensconced in a hospital room at Meritus in Hagerstown. He's getting All. Kinds. Of. Antibiotics! I knew cellulitis was serious stuff and this underscores it.

I came home last night and slept hard. This morning, I realize it's because there wasn't part of me on alert. I could just sleep.

Today I go see Margi, then head up to Hagerstown to see John, then see my cardiologist (who's also in Hagerstown) for an annual check-up, then sit with John and come home late afternoon.

Tuesday, April 16, 2019

John to his group:
> *In hospital getting mega antibiotics for cellulitis in legs. Nice hospital good staff. Be here for a couple of day. At meritus love A visit Room 5301-1*

Wednesday, April 17, 2019

John to his group:
> *Still in the hospital maybe get sprung tomorrow. Legs are getting better after 24/7 antibiotics for a couple of days. Hospital is borrrrrrring. Hi to all the folks at Trillium.*

Thursday, April 18, 2019

John to his group:
> *I think they time the 5 am blood draws, etc, so that at least 3*

people in a row ensure that you do not sleep past 5:15 .

I asked for the star trek instant fix it last week and got a good laugh

nurse just came in and said they are working on discharge papers… freedom beckons

* * *

Freedom! Glad there was a good facility I could go to, and glad I'm home in my own chair at my own desk.

Feeling a good sense of hope for the future today now that the infection in my legs is clearing up. Met a different oncologist at the hospital and will set up a consult with him. He has been treating friends for a number of years and keeping them mobile and active. Feels like synchronicity, we'll see.

Thursday, April 18, 2019

John was discharged this afternoon and is now relaxing in his favorite chair. He's still on antibiotics for a week, but capsules, not shots.

While he was there, one of his pre-retirement co-workers stopped by. She and her husband have both been treated at the cancer center there in Hagerstown. She just goes in for annual checks now. Her husband has been given 6 months to live many times over the past 6 years and he's still doing well.

The oncologist they've been seeing "just happened" (as in this feels a bit more than coincidence) to be the same one that stopped by to see John several times over the 3 days. We're both thinking that a consultation there would be good. That oncologist couldn't say much, but he did say that John's chemo had been pretty aggressive.

I'm feeling hopeful. The first time since all this began.

Tuesday, April 23, 2019

I've had a few days of reprieve from worry. I've treasured them, knowing (like everything) they can be fleeting.

John's cellulitis is diminishing by the day. That's the good news. The not so good news is that he's got increasing nausea and finding it hard to eat (again). I'm suspecting the antibiotic. He doesn't think so cuz it didn't used to bother him. However, this chemo has reset so many of his internal systems. The poor guy isn't getting much of a break and we keep hoping he will.

We have an appt to see Dr. Grant on Thursday for a follow up and a referral to the oncologist in Hagerstown.

Thursday, April 25, 2019

John's feeling a tad bit better today. We saw Dr. Grant and it turns out the antibiotic may well have been causing the nausea, which is the #2 side effect of it.

AND… we've been referred to an oncologist at Meritus in Hagerstown. And not just any oncologist. There are two in that practice that Dr. Grant knows well. So well, that he sometimes gets calls from them to confer about one of their patients. That's not something that happens often. We see Dr. Randoph next Tuesday afternoon. I'm personally relieved that it will be a doctor with English as a first language. I think that was part of the problem we had with Dr. Jafra in Baltimore. The more I think about it, the more I think there was massive miscommunication.

I'm feeling calm and hopeful.

On a completely different subject, I've tried out SunBasket meal delivery. Most of their food is organic and you can choose from vegan, vegetarian, paleo, pescatarian, carb free, and a couple of others. Most of the packaging is either recyclable or compostable. I'm impressed. And the 2 meals I've had were quite tasty.

Monday, April 29, 2019

John to his group:

Kind of getting through a rough spot hear with the endless nausea and fatigue. Doing a consult with another dr tomorrow re treatment options. What I am doing doesn't seem to be doing anything but making me feel worse — which i know is the side effects.

Please keep the prayer and energy coming — this is one of those spots where I can use all I can get. thx

Tuesday, April 30, 2019

John to his group:

Good consult today with a hagerstown dr and more tests, then he may have some ideas for less agressive treatment. If all the side effects from everything I have stuffed into my body for the past 8 weeks would subside, I'd feel a whole lot better.

Hanging in there.

Wednesday, May 1, 2019

We saw the different (and much closer to home) oncologist (Dr. Randoph) today. We'll see him again next Tuesday, after John gets a new PET scan to see what effect the two aggressive chemo sessions had. At that point, Dr. Randoph said we could talk about options and whether it makes sense to switch John's care to him.

This Dr. didn't paint as dire a picture as the one in Baltimore. There is a possibility of an immunotherapy! I need to get a copy of the pathology report from UMMC. I've sent a request to Dr. Jafra's assistant at UMMC for a copy of that report ASAP.

Meanwhile, thrush has raised its nasty head again, so John's taking his lozenges for that. We caught it early this time! So grateful. The hospitalist prescribed 5 refills… and no more steroids! We both hope John won't need those refills.

This doctor just has a better feel to me. I never felt really good about the Baltimore doctor. That feeling hasn't improved. There has been no attempt to check in with John to see how he's doing and they said to give them a call when the infections were gone and John had gained weight. Between the thrush and the cellulitis and the new nasty nausea, he's lost weight. Dr. Randoph is older (I'm guessing early 60's?) and his experience shows.

This new doctor has provided a small ray of hope, which we both needed… badly. It's been a very rough week.

Thursday, May 2, 2019

Today has been a tearful day for me. Not for any specific reason, just lots of little ones, all centered around John.

He's hardly "here" these days. Mostly he's sleeping, like 80% of the time.

And something Dr. Randoph said Tuesday keeps coming back to me. I didn't write it down, and it keeps popping up in my memory. What he said was they look at performance mechanics – as in how active a patient is. The more active, the better the potential outcome. John's not very active and hasn't been for 5-6 weeks. He doesn't have much energy, so he tires easily and he's nauseous pretty much 24/7 at varying levels of intensity. The nausea meds help, but they don't eliminate it.

I'm not sure he even has the energy to take a walk outside. It's allergy season and he's prone to sinus infections. I'm not even sure wearing a simple surgical face mask would help. We have some for when visitors come, since John's immune system is basically shot because of the chemo. Have I mentioned lately that I hate chemo and what its done to John?

He's putting a good face on it, for which I'm grateful, but I'm not sure he's still doing his morning prayers and ritual. He feels defeated to me, which makes sense because of the strong connection between gut health and body/emotional health.

And there's nothing I can really do but be here.

And I'm not a huge fan of chemo right now. Not one f'ing bit!

I keep hearing that being there is "Everything"… not "nothing." Margi said the same thing Tuesday. It's just hard to remember that when I'm feeling helpless. While it isn't as strong as it used to be, my urge to be a control freak is getting a serious smack down cuz this is soooooooooo out of anybody's control.

Sunday, May 5, 2019

John has a PET scan scheduled tomorrow morning (Monday) at 8:30. We'll find out if the chemo helped or not.

The new oncologist asked about a specific test result. I still haven't heard back from the Baltimore oncologist. I DID hear back from his gastro doc in Baltimore. The gastro doc remembers John and he faxed all the results (including the DL-R1, which will show if Immunotherapy will help John) directly to the new oncologist, who we'll see Tuesday morning. I find it interesting that the gastro doc is more helpful than the Baltimore cancer doc, who doesn't seem to care at all about John's health. I keep coming back to us being subject to a "they're just ignorant hillbillies from West Virginia" mentality. It won't leave me alone. Maybe because I need someone to be angry at in general, or maybe because it's real. Regardless, I'm glad we're done with the Baltimore group!

I'm doing a bit better emotionally. Friends have been feeding me tasty homemade food (including Chinese dumplings and cheese soufflé). For some reason, I think I'm "supposed" to be able to handle all this, no problem. Such high expectations. Not a new thing.

I've finished another roll of rugs and I'm now putting on new warp (the strings I weave on) in colors! Since my loom came with lots of warp on it already, this is the first time I'm doing it. So far, so good. It's such a welcome respite.

Going to run errands in a bit, including the Farmers Market.

* * *

Rant alert:

Caregiving is exhausting, no two ways about it. Caregivers are overwhelmingly women. Some research says they contribute over $500B of unpaid labor per year now based on what it would cost to pay someone to do what caregivers do. That doesn't even include the impact on careers, emotional health, physical health, etc. It's a cultural expectation. It's not much different than blaming a patient for their illness, which happens more often than we'll admit.

Somehow, we're supposed to know what to do, when, and remain physically and emotionally healthy. Excuse me?!?

Monday, May 6, 2019

John's getting his PET scan now. Actually, at this point, he's probably waiting for the sugar injection to fully be in his system, then they'll do the 2nd scan to see how the cancer is doing. We'll find out tomorrow.

Monday, May 6, 2019

John to his group:

> *Back for another pet scan today, then meet tororow with dr to see if he has any bright ideas about navigating this mess.*

Wednesday, May 8, 2019

I wrote a post earlier today sharing what's up. FB apparently ate it. Grrrrr.

We saw the new dr yesterday, Dr. Randoph. The news was mixed. The good news is: the spots in his lung and on his back are gone; he has the right something-or-others so immunotherapy is an option. (Dr. Jafra had said there wasn't immunotherapy for this cancer.)

The not so good news is that the tumor is encroaching on both the bottom and the top of the stent. This is the cause of his nausea and why the anti-nausea meds and the pain meds haven't been helping much. Also turns out codeine can cause nausea, so he is switching back to Percocet.

Because of his awful reaction to chemo, that's now off the table as a treatment modality. No tears are being shed. He will start radiation therapy tomorrow (Thursday) for 15 days: 5 days a week for 3 weeks. It's a tiring drive for me on I-70 and there are some ugly drivers. The good news is that his appointments are at 9, after rush-hour is done.

Immunotherapy has a 15-20% success rate, which is better than anything else. It also has very few, if any, side effects. They'll start that once the radiation has shrunk the tumor.

As for me, I'm on a roller coaster. Tuesday's news provided some hope. And it's still a terminal illness. In the course of a day, I'll be experiencing grief, sadness, numbness, hope, anger, frustration, and on it goes.

Cancer is teaching me, in no uncertain terms, that being attached to much of anything is pretty much a waste of energy and time. I get to remember and practice this multiple times a day.

The other thing that happened today was John decided to drive to the pharmacy in Hancock to pick up his meds. He hasn't driven in months! It's a 20 minute drive, one way. Here are our texts:

John – text to Elmdea, 5/8/19, 3:29 pm
I picked up meds a home center. Big adventure for the day.

Elmdea – text to John, 5/8/19, 4:30 pm
Big adventure! Thanks for letting me know so I didn't go over before I came home.

* * *

The reply I wanted to send was *"What were you thinking!?!"* I've talked with a number of friends and my sister about how to address it. John is on Percocet and has been on that or

Codeine for several months. Based on my personal experiences with opioids while dealing with my herniated disc, its aftermath, and back surgery, I know how extended use of Percocet creates confused thinking and poor physical reaction time. I didn't drive the entire time I was taking it for fear of causing an accident. Post surgery and getting off the Percocet was pure delight. I could think clearly again and I had my independence back.

I remember Dr. Randoph's observation about performance mechanics and that more active people had a better chance of having good outcomes from treatment. My understanding was the doctor was talking about physically moving the body by walking, swimming, etc. I'm guessing John took it as meaning getting out of the house. Therefore, he got in his car and drove about 20 miles round trip to the pharmacy. He hasn't driven since February.

I spoke with the social worker at the cancer center and asked if she and the radiology doctor could mention that driving wasn't a good idea right now. I wanted them to be "the bad guys" if John got upset. In the end, I spoke to John myself about my concerns, both for him and for any innocent bystanders if he had an accident, including the potential for a nasty lawsuit, wiping out his estate, if someone decided to sue. I suspect he'll never drive again. I know it will be hard for him. He's used to driving, although he has been doing less over the past few years.

* * *

Mostly right now, I'm tired. Just plain tired. I'm eating, I'm taking my vitamins and anti-depressant and meds. I could probably get more sleep. That said, it's time for me to go to bed. We have to be in Hagerstown at 11:45, for his first radiation session. After that, 9 every weekday.

Wednesday, May 8, 2019

John to his group:

> *Now enrolled as a patient at the cancer center in Hagerstown and will start getting radiation treatment tomorrow. Staff is very helpful and informative. Will do initial 15x radiation and see what happens from there. I am still running very low on energy, so shoot me some extra. Thx!*

Friday, May 10, 2019

Today, I sent a fax to Dr. Jafra in Baltimore. I informed her that we were changing John's care to a Cancer Center closer to home, to better manage John's treatment. I was polite and professional. Burning bridges is never a good idea, as tempting as it can be.

Wednesday, May 22, 2019

It's been close to 2 weeks since I posted. Much has happened, most of it good.

John is now getting radiation, which was rough for about the first week, but now is going well. He still lives on Ensure cuz he doesn't want to rock the boat and make the (now beginning to decrease) nausea any worse. The doctor upped his pain meds so he's now taking 10mg Percocet and that's working. The bestest of best things is… he's doing his morning ritual and prayers, with incense, again! This is major.

I'm learning what respite means and figuring out what I need by way of help. I also learned that grief isn't like depression. It isn't with you 24/7 and it can pop up out of nowhere. I was feeling bad cuz I have many moments of just enjoying my day. The up and down roller coaster is NORMAL! I didn't know that and it's such a relief!

The other good thing is that John is up more/sleeping less. We had a wonderful conversation today that skipped around all kinds of subjects, some very serious, some not… like we used to. It was wonderful. It feels like we've moved into a space of accepting that John's time in this body is limited. Up until now, I think we were trying to wrap our minds around it, while in shock and some denial. For today, in this moment, he's here, he's alive, and enjoying what he can.

Tomorrow I get another spinal injection for my still healing sciatic nerve. Joyce is driving John for radiation and Sally is driving me to Winchester for the injection. Thank you to both of you for helping us out!

On Saturday, I went to part of the annual Druid gathering that happens at The Land Celebration. I got to spend a little time with several very dear friends. John had strongly encouraged me to go, saying he'd be OK here on his own. It was the craft fair part of the gathering and I sold all eight of the rugs I had. I found it interesting that so many people said they would be using them as prayer rugs or in their altar area. I came home recharged.

We see Dr. Randoph on Thursday to see how the radiation is doing on the tumor. We'll also ask for a realistic estimate on John's time left here, knowing that it is just that, an estimate. They've been very clear that what John is receiving is palliative care, not a cure.

I'll post more in a few days re: the oncologist appointment and what I need by way of respite help.

I love you all. Thank you for being here.

Friday, May 24, 2019

John to his group:

This week was about hurry up and wait at the hospital between radiation and infusion sessions. My schedule got mixed up a little, so ended up with 3-4 hour gaps between treatments which meant trying to nap in the car or various lobbies. No real news on whether any of this treatment is helping in a meaningful way – going to have to do more of this regiment and then get retested. I seem to feel better and hope I can stay here pysically for a while at least

Right now we are working through traditional (i.e. insurance approved stuff). If A doesn't work then you can try B. We've spent most of the time trying to get my nausea/pain under control so far. Once this round of radiation is done, we will be headed back for some more trials. Dr. Randoph says I have the right genetic markers for certain immunotherapy treatments to possibly be effective. I'm going to have to do some diving in the deep end of the pool to restore my healing energy connection to the life energy surrounding me. My connections feels weak at the moment, but I am doing that I can to keep the channels open and flowing, so please keep praying for me and sending me positive energy.

Thursday, June 6, 2019

I'll do two posts today: this one, which will be a John update; and another one later which will be a me update.

John is now finished with his 15 rounds of radiation. He cannot do more, given the area that was radiated. Because it's cumulative, he's still feeling the effects: nausea, dry heaves, and (a new one) gas.

A big plus is we are going to the local hospital in a few minutes for his saline IV. It's a whole 5 minutes away instead of almost an hour!!! There's not much I would go there for, but this? This should be fine.

He's now been living on Ensure Enlive and ginger ale for about a month. He's also gained about 5 pounds and his hair is growing back.

We see Dr. Randoph next week for the next bit: 2 rounds of chemo light. In this case, Taxol. He'll get an infusion once a week for three weeks, then one week off, then a repeat and done. After that, he'll be eligible for the immunotherapy. I've mentioned several times to doctors that it seems to be an insurance "thing". No one has corrected me. Yup, we absolutely have death panels in this country. All I'll say about that.

He still mostly sleeps or lies down for most of the day cuz that's just more comfortable.

Oh – Dr. Randoph said the prognosis is unchanged from February, less 3 months, so it's now 3-9 months.

My worry, for this time, is how he'll do on the chemo, even though it is "light".

Tuesday, June 11, 2019

John text to a friend:

I'm still feeling pretty crappy from the 3 weeks of radiation. Been going back to hospital every day for treatment.

Sunday, June 16, 2019

Here's the much delayed post about how I'm doing.

Short answer: I'm doing well.

Longer answer: it feels like I've moved into the next stage of this journey. The first couple of months was shock, grief, denial, more shock, and so on.

Now? I feel like I've adapted. This is the new normal. My schedule is pretty much arranged around John's. I do his laundry; change his sheets; keep the fridge stocked with Ensure Enlive and Ginger Ale so it's cold; make sure he has his cigarettes (Winstons in the red box); make sure his meds aren't running out; pester doctors and whoever for any info, etc. that is needed; get him to the local hospital every day, 7 days a week, (sooooo grateful it's so close!) for about 1½ hours for IV saline and an anti-nausea shot; get him to other medical appointments; and I'm here.

At this point, I feel like I'm basically living alone. Yes, John is physically here, but he's asleep most of the time. When he is awake, he doesn't say much. Part of that is post radiation fatigue, part of it is Oxycodone brain, part of it is I'm not sure what.

I still have times of grief, like when a nurse asked if John used a cane or a walker and a memory flashed of how he looked walking in the front yard sometime before all this started, easy, free, happy.

I still don't need a whole lot of help, I don't think. I'm also realizing I've got things to learn about identifying when I do need help, then asking for it. Most of it is very local.

Julie is helping me with getting the trash out for pickup when she's here, making John's bed (if he's not sleeping in it), and cleaning the house every two weeks.

Sally welcomes me over for tea when I need a different environment; she also would be happy to walk with me; she's also made me some wonderful meals, which froze well.

Joyce has helped with driving John, made me some meals, and helped me with some of my errands.

Anne will soon be baking some things for me and coming over to help me arrange things in "the furniture shed" so there's room in it for the living room couch when it's time for hospice to deliver a hospital bed for downstairs.

Speaking of hospice – I know that's coming at some point. John will start chemo (3/4 dose of Taxol, once a week for 3 weeks) starting June 25. He's getting weaker and weaker, which is no surprise since he hardly moves anymore. Yes, he still gets up and down the stairs about once a day, but he's spending more time sleeping downstairs on the couch. He's existing, trying to make it to the next time he feels OK. I told Dr. Randoph at our appointment last week that John now defines Quality of Life as an hour or two not feeling nauseous. John looked at me and said "I have that." I looked at him. "You do? I didn't know that. You haven't told me." His reply was "I wasn't feeling it so why would I?" Ummmmm...

The subscript I was "reading" at the doctor appointment was that the doctor isn't hopeful. He said that he had been dismayed at the last visit about John's prognosis, but felt better at this one, given what John was saying, which wasn't reflecting a whole lot of what I am seeing. John is determined to make it to the next milestone. His milestones are each treatment option and then the next treatment after that.

Can you tell I'm frustrated? I am. And I have to let it go. His focus is on the next treatment and defeating cancer and death. Yes, the immunotherapy may work for him… and we need to get there first, which is two separate rounds of a different chemo than he had in Baltimore. His first round of the new chemo will start 6/25. Then, and only then, will insurance approve Immunotherapy. Those drugs are apparently quite expensive.

And all this is a way to distract myself from what John is suffering. More and more, it's starting to remind me of how it was before his diagnosis and the stent. The doctor said the upper GI last week showed that the cancer is still hanging over the top of his stent.

OK. This has gotten pretty long. Thanks for hanging in here with me.

Thursday, June 20, 2019

John is only up and awake now for his IV saline infusions. He is also only drinking a max of 2-3 Ensure Enlive a day.

I miss him sooooo much!!! It truly feels like I'm living alone. He's withdrawn inward deeply. I don't pick much up from him these days. Tomorrow I'll call Dr. Grant to see what we should do.

John is hardly getting any nutrition and is weaker and weaker. I think it's time for Hospice. I don't want it to be. I want John back – and he won't be coming back.

John is scheduled to start his next round of chemo next week. We've talked about it and he's not sure he can handle it, especially since Dr. Randoph is on vacation and won't be back until July 5. Part of John wants to get to the immunotherapy to beat this cancer. I get it. I just don't think his body can do it.

Saturday, June 22, 2019

Something has shifted for John.

For the second day in a row, he has declined to go for IV saline.

This past week, he's only managed to average 2 Ensure a day (he needs 4-5). I'd noticed, last weekend, that the supply of cold Ensure in the fridge didn't seem to be going down as fast as it had and started tracking. When I pointed this out to him (yesterday) he insisted he's drunk much more than that and they're piled up in the trash can. I dug through the trash cans. There were 8 empty bottles. The trash goes out every Monday morning. He said he'd do better. Yesterday, he managed 2 1/3 bottles.

We're having some long awaited work done on the house, including new windows downstairs and siding put on. They started with the windows on Thursday. John told me he saw them up on the front porch roof starting to put the siding up. Except the siding hasn't even been ordered yet.

Concerned, I called Dr. Grant yesterday (Friday). He said he's not surprised John's experiencing confusion. He also said "It's possible he's in a transition." When I asked if that meant John is now actively dying, Dr. Grant again stressed "it's possible."

Per Dr. Grant , I'm to monitor John for signs of agitation or pain. If he seems to be comfortable, let him be comfortable.

He's lying down, asleep or ? for about 23 hours a day. It's been gradual, getting to this point.

I'm in tears or on the verge of tears a lot these past days. The last thing Dr. Grant said to me was that there are no right or wrong choices now and to call him if I need him. I have his cell #, so I can. I'm sooooo grateful we have an old-fashioned GP!!

I don't want John to die/I'm not ready for him to die, but is it fair / kind / loving to force him to do things (like going for IV saline) that only make him live longer when there's no cure and all treatments have only made him more and more nauseous and drained more and more of his energy away?

Is it time for Hospice? I don't know. John and I talked about it seriously today. I've brought it up before over the past couple weeks and John was clearly not interested so I dropped it. Now, he's willing to maybe consider it since I told him they would be helpful for me as well as for him. He's not real excited about it but he's willing to hear what they have to say. I've called Dr. Grant for a referral.

What I do know is that John has repeatedly said that, when his time comes, he wants to die at home, in his own bed, with me and Alice (the cat) with him.

I'm not ready for this. I won't ever be.

As of today, he's still doing pretty well. I know what my intuition says and… I've been wrong before. No, he's still not getting much fluid or nutrition, but he's been more here last night and today. I just don't know how to read his health situation any more.

Sunday, June 23, 2019

Elmdea, to John's group
Dear ones,

John is not doing well. Please pray, meditate, journey, think of him.

Radiation kicked his butt, and he didn't have a whole lot left in him to kick. He's eating and drinking less and less and sleeping about 23 out of every 24 hours. He's lost 10 pounds in the past 10 days. He's been living on Ensure Enlive and ginger ale for weeks. Today, he hasn't drunk any Ensure. He did receive a liter of IV saline and has drunk close to a can of ginger ale.

He's experiencing some confusion and the "lines" between past, present, and future are getting pretty fuzzy. One example: he reported watching something with our house maintenance that hasn't happened yet, but will in the next few weeks.

I asked for a referral to Hospice and they came out today for an initial interview. I'll hear more tomorrow.

I'll keep you posted.

Thank you for being John's friends and for loving him.

Sunday, June 23, 2019

A hospice intake nurse came out today. The only potential problem at this point is his IV saline. I made it clear that it's not treatment, it's palliative. I'll hear tomorrow from the primary hospice doctor.

If Hospice doesn't work, they'll sign us up for Home Health, which is nearly the same. The two organizations are in constant contact about their patients so he can be transferred to Hospice when it's needed. I suspect he'll be going straight into Hospice. It's just that the Sunday staff didn't know how Hospice views IV saline.

John elected to go for the saline this morning. While we were there, I had him step on the hospital scale. He's lost 10 pounds in 10 days. This is not good. I'll call the cancer center tomorrow to update them. I seriously doubt they'll want to initiate chemo on Tuesday. John has been using that as his next milepost. I'm not sure how he'll react if it's cancelled. He may just give up, which is mixed for me. I don't want him to die and he needs to be free of his 24/7 nausea, extreme fatigue, and suffering.

John went right to the couch as soon as he got home and has been up maybe 10 minutes in the past 11 hours. He hasn't drunk any Ensure today. The 1 liter of saline and a can of ginger ale is all he's had. I'm not fussing at him about it at this point. He just can't and he's not hungry.

Kate and I are going up to Hagerstown this week to make cremation arrangements because I understand it all works better if it's arranged before it's needed. Thank you, Kerrith, for mentioning that you went with a friend to do the same for your late husband all those years ago. I hope it does help me connect with this next phase. John's memorial will be at a place we both love down in Virginia. The minister who married us will do the service. She's also a very dear friend. She's coming out tomorrow and I suspect we'll cover some of this.

I'll be very surprised if John is still alive this time next week. I know bodies can surprise us, but he has no reserves left.

I did a fair amount of crying yesterday, some today, sometimes nothing at all setting it off. I'm just letting myself feel it.

Yesterday, I found three voice messages from him from a year ago April when Becky and I drove from Phoenix to Seattle, via Cottage Grove, Oregon. I hadn't realized how much his voice has changed! I'm also grateful I didn't delete them.

I've questioned if not pushing him to eat or drink is me failing as a caregiver. I'm rapidly coming to the conclusion that my caregiving role has just changed: it's now to do what I can to make sure he's as comfortable and peaceful as possible.

Tuesday, June 25, 2019

In conversation this morning, I told John this is the hardest thing I've ever done, and I wouldn't be anywhere else.

He asked "Even Sheetz?" and I replied "Even Sheetz." We laughed. The old Sheetz store here, before they moved to their new place, was, erm, a bit dicey. It was a precious moment of John and his wry humor, like before this cancer and the treatments.

Twice during the day, John said "I'm on the road, but there aren't any pull offs. No place to pull over and look."

John's statements about the road are typical of end of life conversations which often feature modes of travel. However, what I don't and can't know is if John has more living to do and experience.

Much has happened the past few days. I've cycled in and out of tears all day, sometimes settling into a place of just seeing all of this as the observer.

To be clear, this isn't about avoidance or denial, but rather seeing all of this as part of the larger play of being human and experiencing all that happens in this world and this consciousness. For those of you familiar with the term, I'm observing samsara.

We got to have a conversation with Dr. Grant yesterday evening re: the wisdom of John going in for chemo today. Dr. Grant's soooo very good speaking with John! He helped clarify some things, like John has questions that need to be answered before going ahead. Dr. Grant also said (paraphrasing) that, at this point, all decisions are good ones.

This morning, after having processed it, John opted to NOT go up to Hagerstown to meet with the strange doctor (since Dr. Randoph is on vacation until 7/5) or attempt chemo. I went ahead and cancelled the first two appointments: today's and the one for next Tuesday.

He was also very happy to give up the IV saline. He said it means he can just relax and not worry about watching the clock.

The hospice nurse came out today and went over all the things hospice can do. John asked for some time to think about it. (sigh) I'm hoping he'll say yes tomorrow. I was so hoping it would be a go today… and I know it will be very shortly. Speaking with the hospice nurse afterwards, just she and I, she said that John is in what they call transition, that he's begun the process of dying.

I was able to make all the arrangements for his cremation using e-mail, my scanner, and the phone. I'm so very grateful for that.

I've tentatively reserved Saturday, July 13 at The Land Celebration for John's memorial.

I've been in touch with John's cousin. Today, I spoke with Mara and, with much relief and gratitude, the two of them will let John's dad know what's going on. They both know him much better and my focus is totally here.

So far today, John hasn't drunk any Ensure, not a sip. I don't think he'll be with us much longer. I think it may be down to days now. Any prayers, remote support for him (and for me) would be much welcomed now.

On a completely different note, I went down to the county offices to get 2 building permits for the upgrade work happening on the house right now, something John very much wants to see happen before he dies. It's happening.

I'm relieved I've been able to get a bunch of this stuff set up before he dies because I suspect it would be incredibly difficult after. I'm going to see what I can do re: his obituary. I really don't want a cut and dried "born, died, parents, wife, children" thing. I want something that reflects who I know John to have been in this life. I've no idea if I'll be able to accomplish that. I know there will be a lot of crying, and that's OK.

Thank you for being here for and with me on this journey. I love you all and I'm so grateful for your presence in my life.

Wednesday, June 26, 2019

I spoke too soon yesterday. He drank a whole Ensure. I know that's still not enough, but hope…

He agreed to Hospice, but only because I say it will help me. He doesn't know what they can do for him and he doesn't want to jeopardize the relationships he has with doctors and pharmacies. I've reassured him that isn't going to happen.

I'm on this intense roller coaster of feeling he doesn't have long to live and hoping he turns around. That's part of why I need the hospice people.

Wednesday, June 26, 2019

Elmdea, to John's group

Thank you for whatever you have been doing. John has been more alert and present these past few days. Please continue if you can.

Thursday, June 27, 2019

A migraine woke me up around 3 this morning, so I sat out on the front porch, in the dark lit by the slow waltz of fireflies and a gradually rising crescent moon.

I've found myself in a spiral of fear that centered around me being wrong and John not dying this week and the grief I've imposed on myself and on our friends and our families. I've delved into this, looking at what was under each layer of feeling.

"What is the feeling under this thought?" I then looked for the feeling under that feeling, and continued until I came to a place of recognizing the very strong negative self-judgment I carry about myself. It's been a life-long companion. I let myself sit with that.

A phrase I've often heard came to me: "your greatest strength lies in your greatest weakness". I think I've found it: from my unrelenting and very harsh self-judgment is my genuine, real, and true ability to be a place where people can share information with me without feeling judged by me. Can I gift that to myself? Maybe, maybe not. And, I'm now aware of it. While I know there are deeper layers, I'm resting in and with this one for now.

Doing this deep shadow work is me honoring the experience John is giving me through his illness and coming death. I don't know how else to phrase it. It's not a conscious or wished for experience. Accepting it and doing the work means I can be more present with and for John as he continues his journey.

As I sit with all of this, I realize there's a strong possibility that much of the family strife that arises around and after death is because it brings up people's shadows and many folk just can't deal with it so they lash out as a distraction. Being in the presence of the terminally ill can bring us face to face with our greatest fear – which isn't necessarily death, but something else.

Some night creature (a cat?) just made some noise in a few fallen leaves. I spoke to it softly. I could see it's movement as a darker darkness in the darkness. That's a metaphor for something.

Looking Back

Five years later, this time seems a blur. So much was going on, all of it so difficult.

To this day, I can see Dr. Grant in our living room saying to me "There are no right or wrong choices now." It lifted a weight from me. I wanted to do everything I could and it was out of my hands. It was in cancer's hands.

This isn't an easy journey for any of us who are caring for a loved one with a terminal illness. In retrospect, the focus on John's comfort was key for both John and me. No more going here and there for this or that treatment. He could now stay home.

I still had much to learn about the resilience of the human spirit and body, John's in particular. The observations of two friends who are energy healers threw me emotionally overboard. One mentioned that John's energy was mostly in his first and second chakras, which are at the base of the torso, and there wasn't much energy in the upper four chakras. They said that when they'd seen this before, that person had only lived another week or so. Another friend said they sensed John had one toe in this world and one toe in the other. I assumed John's death was imminent.

They were wrong. John would be here for another three months. We would have more time, more conversations, more laughter, more love, more learning, more misunderstandings and resolutions. In short: more life to live together. I'm grateful, even though it was painful for each of us in our individual experiences and perceptions.

My healer friends were also right: John was dying. Dying has its own timetable, and it's unique to each person.

The other thing that contributed to my assumption that John would be dying soon was that John kept saying he was looking for "a turnout on the road." I had read that statements about "the road" are typical in end of life conversations which often feature modes of travel.

PART VI:
THE BLESSING THAT IS HOSPICE

Friday, June 28, 2019

I'm doing much better this morning and John is still here and doesn't appear to be going anywhere soon, other than rotating between his bed (upstairs) and the couch (downstairs). He's still not taking in much by way of fluids or nutrition, but he is getting some nourishment in.

The team of hospice nurses will be coming out this morning at 10 to start working with John. At this point, they'll only be coming out once a week, increasing their visits as it becomes necessary, which may be next week or a month(s) from now.

I also now have a phone number I can call 24/7 and I need to pop down to the pharmacy to pick up the Comfort Kit (that's what its called), which I'll only open under the direction of Hospice. It apparently has different meds and stuff that can be used until they can get here if it's an emergency sort of situation.

What I need to remember, among many things, is John comes from a family of long-lived men. His grandfather lived for 98 years, and his father is 97.

A grief social worker from Hospice came out yesterday. I can breathe again. I shared what's been going on with me and It's. All. Normal!

My amped up fears; my conviction that John was going to die this week; my harsh self-judging thoughts; wild mood/feeling swings; has a name: *anticipatory grief,* which is different from grief after a death. Making cremation and memorial preparations contributed to it all.

I get cluster migraines and they showed up this week. They come in clusters because there will be a bunch of days with them, and then many, many without. They usually wake me up at two or three in the morning. This happened three nights this week. While CBD oil helps diminish them, I'm still up for several hours. So sleep deprivation is also adding to everything.

I'm going outside now, to sit in the morning sun, and appreciate the new pale yellow siding that's in the process of being put on the house, something John has long wanted to do and now it's happening.

Saturday, June 29, 2019

John rested well last night.

The hospice nurse came out yesterday and reassured John that Hospice works WITH his doctors, not instead of. She suggested he try something called Haldol to help his esophagus relax. It was in the Comfort Kit, so I got to open it. Interesting stuff in there, most of which I've no idea about. I'm happy to wait to find out. John told her he gets out of breath going up the stairs, so she ordered oxygen, which was delivered yesterday afternoon. It's in the living room, so John can use it when he's lying on the couch.

We finally got the port access out, after much to-ing and fro-ing between hospice and his oncologist, plus an hour at the local hospital as the pharmacy took its time getting the heparin (which seals/protects the tubing in the port so infection doesn't start) sent up. The vein access (or whatever it's called) is still in his body, it's just the external tubing that's been removed.

While at the hospital, a person we'd met at the cancer center in Hagerstown was also there, finishing up an IV saline infusion. He didn't look like he was doing so well either, but had looked fine when we'd last seen him in Hagerstown.

I'm more and more convinced that this whole chemo / radiation thing is still mostly experimental and quite deadly, despite what the medical community says. Yes, it does help some people. I suspect it's mostly those with cancers that are

Stages 1-2, possible Stage 3, but not Stage 4. And even then, no guarantees.

Yesterday was a long, hard day for John and totally wore him out. He had taken one dose of the Haldol and the oxygen for maybe 3 minutes. Later in the day, he wasn't interested in doing either of them because he didn't want to "rock the boat". While I understand that, it frustrates me, which I have to let go. There's so little he can control in his life these days and he needs to feel some measure of control.

* * *

This morning, he's been up for more than an hour! It's been awhile since that's happened. He also seems a tad less confused.

This is so up and down. The next thing to let go of is my desire for consistency and predictability, strengthening my focus on right here, right now.

A friend, who used to work in ER, mentioned that Haldol is used there for extreme anxiety because it quiets the brain. She suggested that it probably also relaxes John's esophagus, and therefore he got better sleep.

A couple of John's friends stopped by or checked in today to see how John is doing. John was sleeping and I didn't wake him. My friend, Anne, stopped by with cheesy biscuits and clotted cream. Yummy. And my tummy is telling me it doesn't like such rich foods right now. I wonder if it's the stress of all this?

Mara has convinced John's father and his partner (Mara's mother) to go down to the beach house, since it's very unlikely that John will have the energy for another visit with his father.

I unboxed my 8" Mirrix Lani tapestry loom. I wonder when I'll get a chance to play with it and start a practice tapestry.

Sunday, June 30, 2019

The Haldol is relieving John's pain

Today was a day of bright light and low humidity.

I learned that ANY treatment for Stage 4 esophageal cancer has a 20% at best success rate. It's also one of the most aggressive cancers at this stage.

Today I know I'll be OK after John dies. I suspect the grief will feel somewhat like I felt after Mouse and Zinnia died – intense for a bit, then dwindling. I'll always be missing him.

Sitting on the front porch, I felt him sitting next to me as he used to. It was comforting. It was also confirmation that he's in my heart in a good and companionable way.

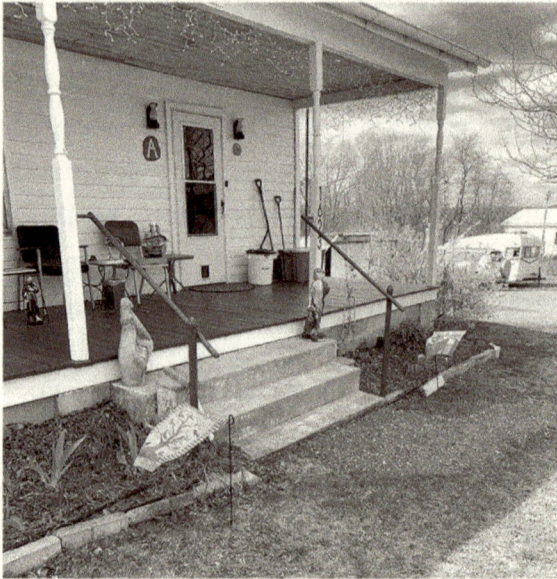

Our front porch, 2019

Monday, July 1, 2019

Out of the blue, with no context, parts of today felt like life used to before John got sick. I was occupied with fairly ordinary things. Grief was minimal. It was there but not overwhelming.

The weather was beautiful today with bright sun and a soft breeze. A plus was that the electrician came and installed A/C on the second porch. Now I don't have to worry about my yarns and fabric getting musty and moldy from the humidity.

I'm getting the strong feeling that there is more for me to explore about my deep self-judgment. It's going to be more than "just deciding" to explore, but I'm not sure what to do at this point. If it's anything like things I've worked on in the past, it will evolve. I explored it a little with Margi during our session today, but most of the time was taken with my doubts about whether I'm really capable of deep intimacy and relationship. It came up because I don't know if I'm doing enough for John. I'm doing what I can, but it never seems enough. "Enough" would be finding some way for him to be healed. That's not in my hands. It's not in his either.

Tuesday, July 2, 2019

Today has been mixed. As all days are now. I'm thankful for being alive and aware.

John got up to hug me good night – and had to vomit.

I learned that Beau killed the black snake that lived near the 3rd porch. I liked it back there. It caught mice. I apologized to its spirit.

I've spent a little time imagining telling Mara and my friends that John has died. Doesn't feel very real, which is fine with me.

And – I don't think John is getting much enjoyment out of life. He's experiencing the kind of death we all dread: long, painful, hopeless.

Wednesday, July 3, 2019

Today, I felt impatient with how long John is taking to die and immediately felt guilty even thinking that. It's a mixture of wanting my simple life back, not wanting to deal with the grief, wanting the man I married back instead of this sick person who is and isn't my beloved John, and just being tired. So, so tired.

I've been reading Final Conversations by Maggie Callanan and Patricia Kelley and how the conversation can occur over weeks, often focused on travel. I'm making some notes for myself about possible cues. My mind is so focused on taking care of John, I might miss them.

In response to me saying that the rain would take the wrinkles out of the dragon flags hanging on the front porch, John replied "There's some sunshine on the other side." It was a cloudy day, a rainy day. I wonder if he's seeing into the Otherworld.

There's a new A/C in the kitchen.

I checked with Hospice to make sure there's enough Haldol until next week when the Hospice nurse comes again. There is. John seemed relieved to know that. And… I'm not sure how much he remembers these days.

Thursday, July 4, 2019

It's been a very up and down day. Even though we never did much on the 4th, I felt very alone. When John gets up, he needs to be by himself to get settled, which takes most of the brief time he's up. I feel more and more like I'm living alone and when I'm not – it's a stranger here, not John.

I've realized that when I became a caretaker, it was literally a role change. Old role (wife) shifts to the background more and more as John becomes sicker and sicker.

I cried, which is good.

Friday, July 5, 2019

The Hospice social worker came out to see me today. Before she came, John asked if he could have some time with her too. I said "absolutely!" John talked of his concern that he really doesn't have much interaction with people anymore because it tires him out so much. She understood. John could only manage about 10 minutes before he was worn out and needed to go lie down.

She reassured me that what I'm feeling and thinking is Very. Normal, including my impatience with how long it's taking John to die. She said it would be unusual if I wasn't. Being a caregiver is overwhelming and this is one of the many ways caregivers respond to the stress. And it's not like there's training for how to be a caregiver. It was a relief. She'll be back next Wednesday to see us both, each with our own hour.

I put in a call to Dr. Randoph, the medical oncologist, as he is back from vacation today. He returned my call around 6. John has wanted to know if there were any options besides chemo. No, there is nothing. I then told Dr. Randoph how John is doing (still losing weight, averaging 2 Ensure a day, some ginger ale, and very tired. I asked him about the chemo session scheduled for Tuesday. He said he wouldn't recommend it. He'd approve it if that was what John wanted. He went on to say to do what I could to provide comfort.

Today I learned that John really is dying. The only thing now is to make him as comfortable as possible.

I'm a little numb.

I don't know what else to say right now.

Saturday, July 6, 2019

I waited until this morning to tell John cuz it didn't seem fair to tell him last evening. He wasn't surprised. I asked him if he wanted chemo. His response was "I have no opinion. I'm still looking for a wide spot in the road."

He'll take this weekend to decide if he wants to try the chemo. I dearly hope he won't, but I told him I would support him, whatever decision he makes. If he chooses the chemo, it will be one of the hardest drives I've ever done.

I'm so grateful for John's presence in my life.

I was talking to my sister Becky on the phone while sitting on the front porch. The blue glass gazing ball rattled and the cement stand it sits in thumped. No wind, no critters. I saw vague shadows. I suspect it's John's kin on the other side letting me know they're here. It helps.

I checked John. He was breathing.

I do that a lot, check to make sure he's still breathing, just a brief pause as I walk by in the hallway as he's sleeping on the couch in the living room. I imagine it's much like mothers checking on their children.

I asked a psychic friend to "see" what she could. She sees John surrounded by ancestors and also Freya or Bridgid there – to welcome his birth there, not waiting for him to die, but to be born. There is no timeline to this.

I asked John if he was afraid of dying. "Yes," he said. "Of losing who I am, losing you, Alice not so much. I'm afraid of pain."

I told him I would be with him when he died.

Earlier today, I told him how grateful I was for our years together and I've felt more loved than ever in my life. "The same," he said.

Ancestors of John, Freya/Bridgid, please, tell me in a clear way when his time is hours away so I can be sure I'm with him. I would like to give him this last gift in his current physical body. Thank you for doing this. Thank you for rattling the gazing ball. Thank you! Thank you!

Saturday, July 6, 2019

Elmdea, to John's group

John has had a hard time finding comfort of almost any kind. At my request, we called in Hospice a few weeks ago and that's helping some. We did that while waiting for his medical oncologist to get back from vacation, which he did yesterday (7/5).

John is currently scheduled for chemo on Tuesday (7/9). Given his physical condition (he's lost more weight and isn't eating or drinking much, and is weak), Dr. Randoph said it could be done, but he wouldn't recommend it. John will be deciding what he wants to do over the weekend. I'll keep you posted.

Sunday, July 7, 2019

John is diminishing day by day, it seems like there's less and less of him here. I just can't imagine what it feels like to know the only way all of this pain and discomfort will end is with death. A cure isn't possible. There was only a 15-20% chance of remission from the beginning, with the chemo, the radiation, or the immunotherapy.

Looking Back

While I said at the time I'd support John if he chose more chemo, I now suspect it would have broken me. I couldn't deny that he was dying. I'd been trying hard, holding on to hope. He had been, too. Words really do fail with these kinds of realizations.

PART VII:
HOSPICE YES, CHEMO NO

Tuesday, July 9, 2019

After thinking about it over the weekend, John let me know yesterday (Monday) he'd decided chemo would only make things worse. It was a hard decision for him because it means there's no more hope for a cure or a treatment that could knock the cancer back even a little.

The hospice nurse changed the dosage on his pain meds yesterday morning. They seem to be helping him rest a little better. She asked if he'd like to speak with a chaplain and told him a little about the 2 who work with hospice. He declined. Then, maybe 10 minutes later, said he'd like to talk to "the navy one." He later told me that talking to a man would be helpful.

Tomorrow the hospice social worker comes. She'll be with John first, then me.

Me? I'm so very, very grateful he decided to not pursue chemo. I had some hard crying yesterday, pleading with Spirit to grant him some mercy and release.

We're getting new siding on the house and Beau, John's friend and one of the folks putting it up, asked John to come out and look at what they'd done today. John obliged. We got out there (slowly) and John turned to me and, very quietly (which is how he talks all the time these days) asked "what am I looking at?" I told him. "Oh." pause. "Yes, it looks nice."

Knowing that he's preparing to go is both a sadness and a relief. I love him greatly… and I'll be grateful that he'll sometime soon be freed of his body and it's suffering. The timing is all in his hands, with his spirit. I've continued to let go and let go and let go – and trust what this process is for his soul and his path. Some days that's harder than others.

Tuesday, July 11, 2019

John had another session with the Hospice Social Worker today. He is, understandably, depressed and perhaps suicidal. I also learned that I am the most important thing worth living for to him.

Earlier, I was feeling angry and enraged. First, I had to go buy him some smaller shorts because he's lost so much weight. Then, because he's feeling suicidal, at his request I had to find all the rifles and pistols and get them out of the house. It turned out there were 7 or 8 rifles and 5 or 6 pistols. Anne will store them.

My fear is that John will live and I'll die from it. I know that's not rational.

Having to find and move the firearms was just one more f-ing thing on my to-do list. And I had to reschedule my periodontal appointment… again!

Monday, July 15, 2019

Aaaand… in my session today with Margi, I hit on a big ol' something I really didn't want to address. So much so that I caught myself thinking, during the session, "OK. I'm done. I don't need to come back."

At which point my internal alarm bells went off. "Oh really? Hmmmm. I've been here before. It's time to absolutely stick with it." And I did and am. It's part of my promise to myself to not waste this "gift" that John's cancer (and all it entails) has provided.

It's breaking me open, and that is a good thing.

Sooooo… I'm off to do a collage/painting of this thing I'm avoiding. I know what it looks like. But my mind has conveniently "forgotten" the details. Tricksy thing, lol. And no, it's not something that needs to remain hidden. I know that for sure, even if I can't remember much else. It's some sort of belief created in my infancy or childhood… I think.

Tuesday, July 16, 2019

I got the collage done. I meditated to get in touch with the feelings, which are quite a mix of contradictions. I'm feeling detached from my life, angry and betrayed. Those are the voices of infant me, who wasn't being touched or held when she cried. I was cold, and no one came to cover me up or warm me.

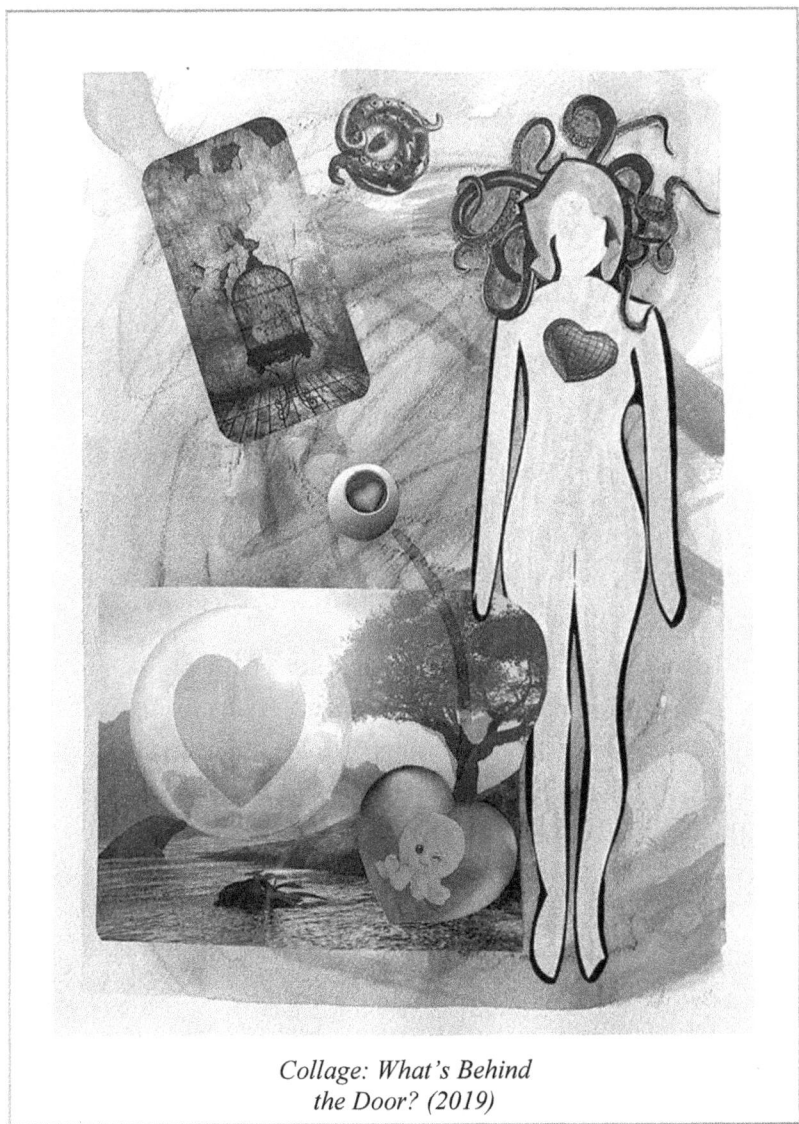

*Collage: What's Behind
the Door? (2019)*

This led me to John. "How dare he die before me!" I want him to be alive and healthy, I'm angry he's sick, and wishing he'd hurry up and die so I can get on with my life. Not a pretty combo of feelings… at all.

The dark tangle behind the figure are the angry, betrayed, scared feelings, attempting to take over, with my heart inside a wire cage. A green arrow points to a murky cage, overseen by an artistic eye. My hope is represented by the heart enclosed in the small white, open ball. The green arrow is pointing to a heart with a fuzzy toy octopus and a rising heart sun.

Wednesday, July 17, 2019

The anger has been building for a while but I haven't recognized it. For some reason I still don't understand, having to buy him new shorts tipped me over the edge. I want my life back: a life where I can do what I want to do, when I want to, without having to worry about John and what he needs. Having to find and move the guns was just adding insult to injury, from that day's perspective.

With distance, I can see it was part of my denial of John's death at some point in the near future. Having to do these things, the denial was replaced with anger.

When I shared this and my collage with the Hospice Grief Counselor, she said it's normal for caregivers to want their lives back, for anger to erupt now and again, and to feel guilty about both of those things. She said there's no reason to feel guilty. It's part of the anticipatory grief process.

Wednesday, July 17, 2019

John, text to his son:

> Lots of brain fog here a late on stuff. Thanks the visit the other day. This is a tough time for everyone to get through. It's all still like dream about half the time. We have our scuffles down the roads. But I lovand want you to have a good life. All for now Dad

Saturday, July 20, 2019

Hospice is a mixed blessing for me. It's a total blessing for John. Hospice and Dr. Grant have figured out a good mix of meds for him. He's eaten some real food (a cookie, several small fruit cups, a piece of zucchini bread) and his stomach didn't rebel. It's been at least 2 months since he's eaten anything solid. He's also up and awake more. He's even gotten on his computer and is also attempting to read a book.

Best of all: his wry sense of humor is popping up again after a long absence. The Hospice social worker and chaplain are helping him start the process of making peace with death as well as addressing any regrets he has.

We've had some good conversations. I'm beyond grateful for them.

For me, Hospice has meant more work. I'm hoping it's just as things get settled and put in place. There have been some days when I. Have. Not. Been. Happy and… they are helping John and that's what counts most.

Anne mentioned that West Virginia has the highest per capita elderly population in the country, followed by Pennsylvania. That, paired with how West Virginia only grudgingly funds anything that could help people means West Virginia hospices are underfunded. Grrrrrr!! And the people we've worked with have been wonderful!

In completely other news, I heard today that a short story I submitted has been accepted into an anthology called *X Marks the Spot*, with a theme of pirates. My story is about cancer: a life pirate. It will be January (or so) before it's published. In the meantime, There. Will. Be. Editing. I'm looking forward to that because I want this story to be the absolute best it can be.

I haven't been doing as much weaving lately. It seems there's so much else I need to be doing. Days seem to slip away. And my looms patiently wait for me to get to them. I'm grateful.

I'm feeling overwhelmed and just plain tired. I forget to eat, which doesn't help. It's not that I don't have food. Kate, Anne, Sally, and Joyce have cooked wonderful food that freezes well and that has helped immensely. But I still have to remember to eat it. This is not a new thing for me. Just saying it here will, I hope, make me more aware.

I am giving myself a treat tonight: I'm going to see *Rocketman* at our quirky local theater. I've heard so many good things about this movie. It will be a wonderful break and John says he'll be fine for the few hours I'll be gone.

* * *

I thoroughly enjoyed *Rocketman*. Powerful story and really well done… and I got a much needed and appreciated break.

Saturday, July 20, 2019

John to his group:

He everybody, Lots of brain fog her a late on stuff. Went through a bad stretch for a while but feeling a litlle better. now under the care of hospice which has been a big help, with getting my meds straighted out. Much better than going to dr all the hospital. and providing some mu ch needed counseling. Getting used to the ideas of dying and how I want to spend the rest of my days is pretty challenging stuff. It's all still like dream about half the time. Thank you all for you continued support. right nwo i am struggling with chemobrain — which is fallout from the chemo. you can't think straifht, typle, read or d anything els like I used to. lots of adaption has to be done, but working on it.

the hospice people are very kind and I really like the fact that I can sit and talk to th enurse for half an our rather than th old chck vitals an nice to see you. my nurse hsa given me some good tips nased on her experiences.

Wednesday, July 31, 2019

Facebook Memories popped up two John things. I don't remember this happening before. On the other hand, I wasn't in this place of grief before.

The first one was that today was John's last day of work in 2012. The next day, he was officially retired. That was 7 years ago.

The second memory was about some peach cobbler I'd made. I'd used Italian seasoned bread crumbs, thinking they were regular bread crumbs. John's comment was "let's just add pepperoni and cheese for pizza." That was in 2015, 4 years ago.

Thursday, August 1, 2019

Something feels like its shifted. No idea what. Beau and Perry are almost done with the upgrades on the house; John had a powerful session with the Hospice Social Worker; and I'm feeling more aware of non-physical presences.

Logged into one of the games I play on my iPad. The first thing that came up was *"John is an incredible man. Someone should make a documentary about him."*

Wednesday, August 7, 2019

John's been enrolled in Hospice for a little over a month now and it's made such a difference! His pain is better managed and he's even been reading a book and "doing" some e-mail. This is huge. The past few days have been slower for him, not reading, emailing, not drinking as much Ensure or Ginger Ale. I'm not freaked by this. Things ebb and flow with this.

What's helped me most is a mindset I've created for myself: John has 3-6 months. Is that his current prognosis? I have no idea. I don't think anyone really knows. What it does for me is take me out of hyper alert mode, which is a very good thing. I know my mind has made this prognosis up and it still works.

Paradoxical things, minds can be. What's even more interesting is how, back in February, when his prognosis was 6-12 months, or more, I was totally freaked out. Of course. It was new. I guess I've come to terms with this new reality: John has cancer. He will die sometime soon. He's alive right now. My life has changed, and it will change again, and again, and again, as it always has.

I'd asked John if he would consider going to the Hospice in-house facility so I could take some time to go visit my mother (who's 91). It's been more than a year and I usually fly out to Phoenix twice a year to see her and my sister, Becky. I was also really clear that if it doesn't work for him, then it doesn't, and I'll be OK with that. He suggested a 2 day trial run, so he can see what he thinks. He mentioned that it might be nice because he could be somewhere else and meet some people for a change. The current plan is that he'll do the trial run Sept 9-11. If that works well for him, then he'll return Oct 16-22 so I can fly to Phoenix, stay with my sister and see my mom.

Work on the house is almost done. The whole house now has siding and looks like everything was planned, instead of tacked on here and there. Lots of neighbors have commented on how great it looks. There's a new roof over the middle porch (my weaving space) so I don't have to worry about rain and leaks any more. I can now open the garage door on my own… easily! There's a roof over the back door, and many other things John wanted to have done for me for when he's not here anymore. All that's left are the two windows in our shared office space (Pella keeps screwing up the order), the upstairs hallway ceiling, and this and that small things. I keep thinking Spirit has something to do with this, to keep John here a bit longer.

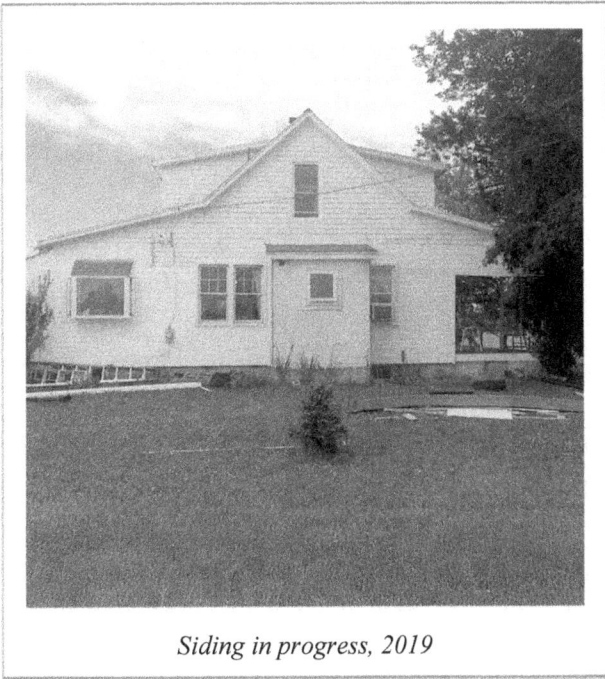

Siding in progress, 2019

Today, I get to finally meet with an anticipatory grief counselor from Hospice, here at home. I don't have to drive there (45 minutes)! I don't feel like I really need it right now and… I know there will be times I do.

Sunday, August 11, 2019

Elmdea, to John's group:

Hospice is continuing to be a huge blessing! Their ability (and knowledge) with pain meds is helping John be more comfortable.

He's been able to read a little and is now doing some limited email and social media.

He's continuing to work with the social worker and the chaplain, who both support and challenge him.

I'm working with an anticipatory grief counselor, which is helping me, and therefore John.

Monday, August 12, 2019

Over the past week/week and a half, John's been drinking about 2 Ensure a day. When the Hospice nurse asked this morning about his hunger, he said he drinks a shake when he is. This from the man who used to say he was born hungry and had to eat something every few hours.

He started a time-release pain med last Friday, so that's making him sleep a bit more.

And I've been getting "messages". It started around August 1. Things like waking up to the smell of coffee brewing and thinking, *wow, John's fixing coffee. He hasn't done that in awhile. I wonder how it will sit?* And just enjoying the smell. I get up and, nope, he hasn't made coffee. Later that same morning, an owl flew over my car as I was driving to Winchester. It's rare to see owls flying in the daytime. They can portend a death, when seen like that.

A week ago Friday, I suddenly "knew" I needed to get the 2018 taxes to the accountant. We'd filed an extension, so I have until October 15. And the knowing was definite. So I got them done and to the accountant last Friday.

Last night, Miz Alice (the cat) was doing a quiet meow, a lot. But she didn't really want to get on the bed. Later, I got up to pee and she was sleeping on the marble surface of the bedside table, something she hasn't done since Mouse died over 2 years ago. She's been really clingy today. When we adopted her, the only thing they could tell us about her was that she was a surrender and her former owner had died. She may (or may not) be picking up on something. I wondered if John had died and decided to wait until morning, to sleep before my world changed. John was OK when I got up.

I've been saying to myself he has 3-6 months. It feels like it's time to revise that to 1-12 weeks. His dying is feeling very real. Not that it wasn't before, but it feels "real-er" now.

I'm not freaking out, like I was back in July. I seem to be making peace with the reality that he will be dying, sooner rather than later, while being (mostly) OK with not knowing when. I'm really understanding, at a gut level, what people mean when they talk about a death being a relief and a blessing for the person who died. Not that John isn't having good moments, but he feels less and less present.

Having written all of this, he's turned around before and he might do that again. I'm not trying to make a case either way. Just noticing.

Thank you for reading my sort of stream of consciousness / processing post here.

Two of his kids are coming to visit today, so part of his bequests will also be done. It's so very, very real right now.

Tuesday, August 13, 2019

I'm more than a little pissed right now. Two of John's kids were coming to see him this afternoon (and to pick up the nearly new riding mower he's giving them). Last minute, I get a "so sorry, things got busy, we won't be there" message from one of them. They message me because John's notoriously bad at getting voice and text messages.

John's doing his work to make peace within himself and with them. I'm being very, very good and not saying anything to them. But boy would I like to, so it's probably good I won't. There's soooooo much I could say.

Rant over – and thank you for being a safe space for me to rant.

Update: I just spoke to John. He's disappointed and said they were just being who they are, then went on to say "I've done what I can." The way he said it makes me think he's done trying. He reached out. They didn't reach back.

* * *

Update: they're coming Sunday morning about 10:30! I'm soooo grateful. I have a gut feeling they'll actually be here. Forces are at play.

Wednesday, August 14, 2019

Today I keep feeling like everything with John and his cancer is unreal. That it isn't really happening. I know it is, and it feels so unreal/surreal.

I'm fully realizing that, as a culture, we are too sheltered from death. My sense of un-realness isn't denial so much as acknowledgement of how very real this process is I'm witnessing in John, a diminishment, a fading, all while he's still very much alive, laughing sometimes, enjoying sitting in the sun, making an occasional wisecrack, falling asleep in his chair.

Friday, August 16, 2019

I'm in a bit of denial again. John is drinking 1 Ensure a day (for 4-6 days? I quit keeping track a while back) and 1½ ginger ale a day. That's 620 calories a day.

Beau, one of the guys who's been doing work on the house, mentioned that John didn't look as good as he did 2 days ago, when he saw him last. He and John are good friends, so Beau knows how John should look.

I'm soooo not ready for this next stage. I'm still sticking with my 1-12 weeks, but it's not feeling very realistic today. I've zero idea what it is.

Can I go disappear and come back when it's all over? I know I won't and can't… no more words…

Saturday, August 17, 2019

John hasn't drunk even part of an Ensure today. Earlier today, I asked how his day was. He said it was a little difficult and his stomach feels like there are rocks in it.

He's wanting more information about what happens, physically, as end of life gets closer. I told him that people eat less and less because their digestion just isn't up for it. I added that it might be the cancer. He didn't seem surprised or upset. His feet are also starting to swell, so his circulation is not as strong.

I still feel slightly removed and also making further peace with the fact that his body has begun its process of shutting down. Some tears today, some rage that this is happening, some resignation, gratitude that 2 of his kids are coming out tomorrow and the third is coming on Tuesday. Words are inadequate to describe what I'm feeling / experiencing.

Tomorrow is my birthday. Our small local theatre is showing the new *Lion King*. That will be my birthday present to myself. Anne, Donna, and Sally are joining me.

As you all know, there was a time not long ago when I needed someone to be here when I wasn't. John didn't need or want that. He still doesn't. I have a sneaking suspicion he'll exit this life when I'm not physically near him because that's who he is: a very private person who has trusted me with seeing and sharing so much more of himself than he does with anyone else. I've been so blessed and I'm grateful. In this moment, I absolutely know the love will remain, even when he's no longer embodied. We've done this life dance together many times and we will again.

Saturday, August 17 , 2019

Right now, it's important to not nag John about eating as I notice him eating less and less. It's part of the comfort I can provide because 1) John won't feel bad / angry / frustrated about not being able to eat or 2) try to force himself to eat and get nauseous or experience some other discomfort / pain.

John's body is having difficulty processing food, even Ensure. It's part of the end of life process. The other thing is that as the disease has progressed, who he is has changed and continues to.

Sometimes, it feels like I'm living with a stranger, who I still love because of who he used to be. That "old" him peeks through now and again, but less and less frequently as he gets closer to death.

My grief counselor says it can be hard for us caregivers to make peace with the decreasing need for food because "we need food to heal and be strong" and at end of life, that isn't part of the picture. I'm having to learn this, grateful for the support from in-home Hospice. I'm not starving John. His body literally can no longer process food very well.

Another thing I've learned is that my primary relationship with John changed sometime in these past months. While I'm still his wife, that's fallen WAY in the background. My primary role is caregiver. It's a hard switch. I remember the last hug I got from John, my husband, and where we were standing: near the radiator in the kitchen.

I remember it now because, looking back, since then I've been more caretaker than wife. He's been more the cared for than husband. Because we've had to be.

Sunday, August 18, 2019

The two kids made it… on time! John got to say what he needed to say to them. I'm not sure how much they took it in, but it was said and it's now theirs to be with / do with as they will.

Change of topic: I need to be clear. I have no idea how long John has left. The early end of life "stuff" can go on for weeks or months. What I've been doing / sharing with all of you dear friends is my process of coming to terms with it. While miracles do happen, I don't think they will here. His daughter asked him today if there's any chance this could turn around. John said "No." That in itself says what needs to be said. He's making his peace with what he can with the time he has, which none of us knows with any certainty.

John is barely getting 1 Ensure Enlive down a day.

His right foot is swollen and, tonight, when I hugged him, it felt like there's a lump at his left waist.

The thought before I went to bed was "kiss him goodnight. There's a chance he won't be here in the morning."

Thursday, August 22, 2019

John to his father:

Dad, thank for your honest feeling about my canacer. It is a hard thing to get your mind around. Sometimes I cry whe i don't want to, otherimes I can't cry when I really want to.

Nonr of the orthodox mrthods of tratment seem to hlp much, so I guess from here on we just seewhat happens.

I'm sorry to take so long to get back to you — I was trying to compos a brilliant resonse, but ended up just just my togue in knots.

thanks you again fo yor honesy and support.

Saw all tree kids this eek. C and K on sun, mc and tues. they all seem to be getting by in their own fashion. MC hs a warehoue jobs putting boxes into boxes, K starts school this weej, and C is looking for a rgulart job as well as doing yard work..I gave them my riding mower.

I amd still working with hospice, whci continues to be a big help. We are focussing now on looking at and repairing important relationships. The issue of how much time I have left is also being lookied at. We are still fooling around wirh my meds reying to get a balance of pain and nausea relief and not toofuzzy headed.

sorry my typing is bad today. Anyhow, more later. Are there any MLB baseball teams worthe following right noW?

love P

Friday, August 23, 2019

John's drinking a little more Ensure, not much. On Monday, I asked the hospice nurse how long John had — days or months. Later, I told John he had 2-3 months. It hit him like a ton of bricks. He was silent. I apologized. It took until Wednesday for him to accept my apology and he said "think before you speak." I was enraged and stayed that way until Thursday. I was lying down, resting, and realized I had a choice: I could keep the rage or let it go. The rage served NOTHING! I let it go. It was that easy. I was (and am) amazed.

This whole experience brings up soooo many emotions, many of which I know are covers for something deeper. And I don't have much energy for going deeper these days.

Sunday, August 25, 2019

John to his group:

Hello to all my friends..thank you for your conitnued prayer and support, every little bit helpd. not a very good week, my body id acting up and we are plating with the meds again. Highlight of te week waw getting to wee a 3 of my kids for brief visits — which is all I can nandle at the moment. I am not unudergoing any active treatment becauwse therre really isn;t anyhing avaialbl.e except a round of heavy chemo drug and my reaction to thid kind of drug last time roi=ound was just jast awful giving the fact that I have e limited time left, i chose not not to spend it sick from chemo. we finally finished a 6 week home improvement projct — windows, roof repair, siding, and the hose looks great. Meta phycial struggle of the week — I waass initially given the stndard 6 month, a year, maybe more. 6 months have passed, so te remainder if in the hands of the gods. We will just have to wait and see. love and thanks to all for your support.

Tuesday, August 27, 2019

Last week was a really hard week for me. Mostly because the emotional impact of this has, I believe, finally caught up with me.

The work on the house is finally done, but the last bit was, ermmmm, messy what with drywall. I now have an upstairs hallway that needs to be repainted. That is on a far future to-do list. While the guys said they'd cleaned up after themselves… not. The upstairs ceiling is repaired now, however.

I got 3 years' worth of cardboard recycling out of the 3rd porch. It took 2 trips to the recycling center. Fire hazard greatly reduced.

I asked for, and received (and needed) a lot of hugs last week.

John and I had a mis-understanding. We've rarely had them in our 8 years together. It's resolved, but it was painful and hard.

Today, I cancelled my physical therapy appt because an adjustable bed was being delivered. "Adjustable" is the Hospice euphemism for a hospital bed. John requested this on Monday (yesterday). He's no longer able to go upstairs because he's now so weak he's afraid he'll fall. He was also having a really hard time getting up off the sofa, where he's been sleeping. After the delivery and a brief "test nap" he said he's glad it's here. He feels safer.

To get that bed here, however, I had to get the Queen sleeper-sofa moved. That puppy is VERY HEAVY!!! A friend came through. While I'd planned on storing it in the furniture shed, that was just too far away for them to carry it. It's now sitting on the front porch with a clear plastic slip cover over it. It looks very West Virginia.

The other problem this week is water pressure. The plumber came over yesterday and we thought it was fixed. It's now worse and he can't get back here for quite a few days. I think I've identified all the problems, but... in the meantime, there's not enough pressure to take a shower. I may need to go to the gym and use their shower.

There are days now when John looks a little yellow, which would be his liver. My understanding is that, given how little nutrition he's taking in (still averaging 1 – 1½ Ensure a day and @ 20 oz Ginger Ale), organ failure is inevitable. Timing remains as it always has: unknown. Absolutely and totally unknown. Which, in truth, is the same for all of us.

Oh – I almost forgot. John has pretty much decided he needs to change his DNR form. Right now, it says he wants CPR. For those of you who don't know, our neighbor's father-in-law died last week. They couldn't find his DNR so the EMT's had to do CPR, even though his body was already cooling. In the absence of a DNR, they are legally required to do CPR to try and restart the heart, at least in the state of West Virginia. Unknown to me, that information apparently had an impact on John. I think that, tomorrow, when the hospice social worker comes to see him, he'll be filling out a new DNR saying no CPR. I'm grateful.

Meanwhile, I get to watch this wonderful man diminish, suffer, have good moments, have despairing moments, have dry heaves, sleep a lot. As of last week, I've begun praying for mercy for him. I don't know what else to do. Yes, being here for him is important. We talked about that, and how exhausted I am. He's worried about me. I told him the only way I know to solve what I'm experiencing is to stop loving him, which isn't going to happen. He got a wry grin and nodded his head. I do have some other things I'm trying to pull together to support me and my physical and emotional health.

Thank you, dear ones, for all of your support, your love, your you-ness.

Wednesday, August 28, 2019

For some reason, the whole thing about John driving to Hancock, back in May, came up for review today. I over-reacted. After that brief trip, John knew he didn't have the focus or the energy to drive any more, but I couldn't see that. I still saw him as the essentially strong and healthy man I'd always known, who could still make fairly sensible decisions. Denial was fully alive and present in me.

Thursday, August 29, 2019

Ummmmm… things are changing. On top of everything else, John now has shingles on the top and left side of his head., the side he sleeps on. He said his hair hurts. Fortunately, the pain meds he's on are helping with the pain. Hospice has ordered lidocaine cream which the pharmacy will have late tomorrow morning.

I called Dr. Grant this morning to see if I can get shingles from John. You can't contract shingles from shingles. You can contract it from chicken pox or, as in John's case, if your immune system is compromised AND you've had chicken pox. Then the dormant virus becomes active. I'm doing what I can to keep my immune system in good shape.

When he shuffled to the bathroom earlier, his balance was pretty dicey and his left ankle seemed like it wasn't strong enough to be straight. He's trying out the walker.

Things aren't looking good and… I now know he could continue for weeks longer.

Pray for us please.

Friday, August 30, 2019

This is what say to myself each day now

At the end of the day,
Remind yourself that you did the best you could today,
And that is good enough

John is noticeably weaker. He continues to be very unsteady when he walks. I can see it won't be long before he's bed-bound. His left ankle looks like it wants to fold in on itself sometimes. And his balance. He laid his cane on the bed and almost fell over. It's now come to the time when, if I'm going to be gone for very long, I'll need to have someone here in case he falls. Not so they can get him up. While he's lost probably half his body weight (he started around 290), he's still too heavy for one person. For all of us: call Hospice, see what they want to do, and make him as comfortable as possible on the floor.

I'm not sure what we'll do about him wanting to smoke a cigarette. I really, really, really don't like cigarette smoke in the house! A particularly sad thing I witnessed today was him having difficulty getting the Bic lighter lit. He complained that they were making the lighters harder to use. He's gotten that weak.

I continue to pray for mercy for him. The suffering is dragging on and on and on. He's experiencing the kind of death none of us wants: lingering illness, progressive weakness, mind dulled by very necessary pain meds.

* * *

Sitting down to dinner, the thought comes that maybe I should check on him, make sure he's still breathing. No. If he isn't, it won't hurt to wait until after I've eaten because the world will change for me when he's not breathing this air anymore. So I eat dinner. And he comes shuffling out to go to the smoking porch. My world stays the same for a while longer and I'm glad.

At the same time, I pray for mercy, that his suffering can cease. There is no getting better, only getting worse, and worse, and worse. No end until the end of life, then peace. May he have peace, please, may he have peace.

* * *

His poor body can't go on much longer. It feels like the shingles is one challenge too many, on top of the cancer.

To see him walk, and how his legs will twitch/jerk, then go to tip-toes. Like the message isn't going well from brain to muscle, or his leg muscles are spasming. He's going to fall, at some point. Then I'll call Hospice for help getting him up.

Please, God, let him die while he's sleeping. Please. Enough. Please. I ache for him, for his suffering. For how his own cells have mutated and are now consuming him from the inside out. So much of his life has been a challenge, and now his death is, too.

* * *

I don't know how many times a day I pause and look at him as he sleeps, waiting to see if he's still breathing. I've been doing this for months. I'm becoming practiced. I just checked again. Sometimes, there's a space between breaths and I feel myself getting tense. Is this it? No, not this time. And feeling the relief, knowing he's still here.

Such a roller-coaster of wanting him to be free of this body and its pain, and wanting him to live, to still be here.

* * *

I got the lidocaine cream today, but he hasn't wanted it yet. An aide came by this morning to give him his first ever sponge bath. He said he feels better for being cleaner. I'm grateful for that.

I'm treasuring the moments: brief hugs, laying his blanket over him when he gets in bed, bringing him his ginger ale (with only 3 ice cubes, because the 8-9 he was using now makes it too cold), giving him a kiss on the cheek. Any one of these could be the last… or not.

There is a large quietness/silence within me that's sharing space with grief and love, tears, and hope for mercy for John and his suffering.

Saturday, August 31, 2019

John is doing a bit better today. His walk is steadier, he's a tad stronger, the shingles is less painful (we got the antiviral soon enough to have a good result).

In meditation this morning, I "got" that his soul has more it wants to accomplish in its current body. I'm here to continue supporting and holding the space for him to do that.

Yes, it's very hard sometimes and sometimes it's easier. There's no place I'd rather be right now than right here, right now.

Sunday, September 1, 2019

Is it just me, or do other caretakers experience this, too? As John gets nearer to end of life, it's almost like he's a stranger, both physically and mentally/emotionally. There are (very) brief moments when the man I love shines through, but mostly he's not really "here" anymore. It's not that he seems to be connecting with the spirits of his loved ones, it's more that he just doesn't have the energy for much of anything anymore.

At the same time, my love for him is deepening, more than I thought it was possible to love and I already love him soooo very much. Now it's more.

Tuesday, September 3, 2019

During meditation, I met John's alcoholic higher self who fragmented off decades ago. He was in a hazy dark corner.

With help from his mother (who died 10 years ago) and Bridget, I brought the two aspects of his higher self together. I requested that his mother and Bridget assure John that "he" doesn't disappear when he leaves this current body. I left them with Bridget, who is assisting the integration.

Thursday, September 5, 2019

I'm going places I didn't anticipate in my session with the hospice anticipatory grief therapist.. She observed that it's actually my heart guiding me now, rather than my thoughts. She also commented that when I deflect (laughing, changing the subject, etc.) it's my mind saying "too much feeling."

I wouldn't have deflected so much today if so much heart stuff wasn't coming up.

John is weaker and weaker, sleeping more and more, interacting less and less. He's back down to one Ensure a day. He is more haggard and more yellow. His kidneys and his liver are not happy. I don't know how else to describe it. He's sleeping more, interacting less, more and more inward, and more jaundiced. It's painful to witness.

What I'm remembering now is something my father taught me after he died: that no matter how messy or awful someone's life looks to me, it doesn't mean they aren't fulfilling their soul's purpose for this incarnation.

Earlier this week, I remembered this, and put two and two together. I've been supporting John's decisions, regardless of my feelings or thoughts about them because I don't know what his soul's journey is for this life. I "got" that at a much deeper level this week. John hasn't had an easy life. He isn't having an easy death. These past eight years with me have, I sense, been some of the gentlest of his life. While witnessing this cancer eating him alive isn't easy, there's a more peaceful place within me, trusting that he, too, is fully living out his life purpose, regardless of how it looks to me as witness and as one who loves him deeply.

Yes, I often find myself in tears of grief, more often now than before. I continue to pray for mercy for him, and for me.

John told me today that he doesn't think he can manage doing a test run at hospice and apologized to me. I told him I understood and I agree. I don't feel anymore that I can be away from him for a week to visit my mother. I just don't. We're both trusting ourselves. For me, it's another acknowledgement that John's physical death is nearer than I want it to be, whenever that is, which could still be many, many weeks.

Tonight, for the first time ever, John asked me to tuck him into bed. I felt honored and privileged to do so, feeling great tenderness and love for him. I tucked him in, carefully, lovingly, tenderly, rubbing his back gently. I snuggled against his neck and said "I love you."

The end of his days is approaching more rapidly now.

Friday, September 6, 2019

I came home from my semi-annual appointment with Dr. Grant. Alice was shaking and seemed to need reassurance. She IS John's cat.

Monday, September 9, 2019

John fell in the kitchen at 3:30 this morning, coming back in from the inside smoking porch. He wasn't hurt but he was too weak to get up by himself. I called Hospice and they asked me to call 911. I called and told them "no siren." They came and I made sure they saw his DNR and told them he's in Hospice and he doesn't want to go to the hospital. They helped him get back in bed.

I've asked Hospice for a volunteer today to sit with him because I have my last physical therapy appointment and then one with my therapist. The Hospice nurse was already scheduled to be here at 10 today, so that's good.

I'm not sure how I'm doing right now. Teary. Stunned but not surprised. I was in bed, but it had been a restless night. I heard a sound that wasn't normal so I came down to investigate and there he was on the kitchen floor. I didn't panic. I made sure he was ok and as comfortable as possible and called Hospice.

I don't know what else to say right now. I'll keep you posted.

I'm going to see if I can get some more sleep, in the recliner by his bed.

I'm working on lining up caregivers for when I'm out of the house. He really can't be left alone anymore. He needs help moving about.

As for his cigarettes, I think at this point it's more the habit of the action cuz I've noticed he isn't inhaling all that much. Not sure the nicotine patches will work because his skin is getting really paper-y. The gum might, but I'm betting it will tire him out. But I'll offer it.

Monday, September 9, 2019

(late evening)

It's been a loooooong day.

I "slept" in the recliner and my sciatic nerve Is. Not. Happy! It's been many months since it felt like this. Between taking care of John on the floor (and being careful) and the recliner, I've set that healing back. Oh well.

The Hospice nurse came at 10. From what I can figure out from what he told her, he came out of the smoking porch, turned to close the door, lost his balance, fell back against the wall and slid down it, coming to rest against the radiator and skinning his left side along his ribs on his way down. Nothing broken or cracked. But his side hurts. It is, of course, the side he usually sleeps on, and still is.

The nurse said it will be at least 2 days before he gets back to "normal". I asked her after, just she and I on the front porch, what percentage possibility there is of that actually happening, realizing that there's no real predicting. While she didn't hazard a percentage, for the first time ever, she went over the sort of things he's likely to experience. They were all what I've read are end of life things – as in the immediate precursors to the actual end of life stage. And… his prognoses, in essence, remains what it's been: days to weeks, or more.

He's incredibly weak. He's restricted to the living room for now, and the bed. He's so weak that, when he lies down from sitting up on the edge of the bed (for meds, to drink some ginger ale, use the urinal) he can almost get one leg up and can barely move the other. I don't see this improving a whole lot, between muscle atrophy from not moving much, serious lack of nutrition, and the cancer eating away at him.

Many tears (but not in front of John) today. This is all just getting realer and realer. Not that it hasn't, it's just more imminent, rather than "out there."

I have 2 caregivers lined up for the next 5-7 days to be here from 11 pm to 7 am every night except tonight. I'm hoping to get a 3rd caregiver, just in case.

Tonight, I'm sleeping in the kitchen on a tried and true, dependable old army air mattress. It works. I inherited a little hand bell my maternal grandmother would use to "call" my grandfather when she needed help when she had Fallopian tube cancer. It's now sitting by John for him to use. I had no idea it would relive its previous use. There's an electronic, wireless one on the way (thank you Amazon Prime) so I can, for example, be in my studio and he can still get my attention.

Tomorrow, a bedside commode and a transport chair will be delivered. A transport chair is a narrow wheelchair with wheels on the feet, instead of the big ones on the side. Thank you, Hospice!!

I'm looking forward to, hopefully, getting some sleep tonight. We'll see. I'm so tired, now physically as well as emotionally. And… John is here at home, as he wished. He's told me many times today "I love you." In the past, he's rarely said that, but always showed me with his actions. I've told him many times today that I love him. At one point he said "I'm glad somebody here does."

Wednesday, September 11, 2019

John is getting weaker and weaker. It's been two days since his fall and he hasn't returned to how he was before. He can barely stand any more. He's declining quickly and it could still be weeks, or more, before he's ready to go to his soul's next adventure. Something in his eyes has changed too. Even though they are quite yellow (jaundice), they are also clearer in a very different way, like he's "seeing" more? I'm not sure how to describe it, but I can definitely see & sense the difference.

I'm feeling soooooo supported right now! I have 5 caregivers, working different days and hours, covering 16 hours a day, 7 days a week. What has been totally unexpected is how they are caregiving *me*. It didn't even occur to me that that would happen, too. And it all came together in about 24 hours. John fell Sunday, I realized Monday I now officially needed help caring for him, and the first caregiver started working last night (Tuesday). Julie referred a friend to me and she worked today. By the end of the day, she'd told me that, if someone else falls through, to give her a call. There are 4 people in her family, including her, who can fill in and help, and they're only maybe 10 minutes away.

I'm burning some incense in the living room every now and again. It's one John likes, so it's soothing for him. I'm not playing music, since his hearing is so bad it just sounds like muddled noise.

Yesterday, I woke him up because the bath aide was here. He opened his eyes and said "who are you?" I said something like "you know who I am." It was only later that I realized he truly didn't know. I think he's begun to travel both worlds. I also think his brain isn't working as well. There have been several times over the past few days when what he says doesn't match up to what has happened.

In their own ways, the Hospice people are now letting me know that John has entered the phase before death. He can be here several weeks, or days, or hours. No telling. I suspect it will be longer because he hasn't quite made peace with his own dying yet. I soooo hope he can. I can sense loving spirits, waiting to greet him and guide him when he leaves this poor, weak, hurting body.

And I cry a bit. I sleep a bit. I feel normal for a bit. I feel brain mushy pretty often. I lay beside him and hold him for a bit. I treasure that so much.

John had a session with the Hospice Chaplain and, after, the Chaplain indicated he'd like to speak with me. We stood out in the sun in the yard as he told me that John has been seeking grace and, today, has reached it. That John is now at peace. I'm so grateful.

Thursday, September 12, 2019

John wanted something "3 ingredients. A, B, C" was as close as he could come to describing it. I finally figured out it was one of his meds.

Friday, September 14, 2019

Elmdea to John's father:

John is resting well, but is very, very tired. I asked him if he wanted to see you or if he'd like me to send you another email. He said "not right now". It's my sense that he doesn't want you to see him like this. In addition, his pain meds make it difficult for him to think and process right now.

Re: the shingles. We thankfully caught them early enough that there's very little pain at this point.

Sunday, September 15, 2019

It's been a week since John fell. A hard week. A week of absolutely knowing the Divine is orchestrating so much. A week of great grief, of deep love, of learning to receive and let others "do," a week of dread.

He's stopped eating. He drank ½ an Ensure on Friday, none since. He's still drinking some Ginger Ale and some water. He can hardly sit on his own. This master storyteller can't find the words for simple things he wants.

Through it all, he remains my chaos coach. The living room is half dis-assembled, bit by bit. I've never liked smoking in the house. But how could I tell him "no"? It's one of the few pleasures he has left. So now I burn incense to help mask the cigarette smoke. I also had drawn a very firm line: I'm NOT dealing with his poop. Until today. We both survived.

I have caregiver coverage 24/7 now and I'm grateful John set things up so it's covered. He's now on liquid pain meds because he was having trouble swallowing his pills. Tomorrow, he'll get a catheter, at his request.

What I absolutely hadn't anticipated? Somehow, amidst my grief, his suffering, the true horror of how cancer destroys a body, I'm even more in love with him. I don't know how that's happened, but it has.

I've let him know it's OK to go. I can feel him moving closer to the Summerlands/Otherworld. I'm reminded again of the paradox of how strong and how fragile these human bodies are. While I doubt he'll make it through this next week, he's surprised me many times before.

I don't know what else to say. Please pray for peace for each of us.

Wednesday, September 18, 2019

(Very early morning)

John is restless tonight. I sat with him for a bit. My sense is it's really sinking in that he will never feel better. I can't even imagine what he's physically feeling in his body. He now has a catheter and can't control his bowels. He was ashamed when he asked me to buy adult diapers a few months back.

His last "food" was ½ Ensure last Friday (five days ago). He still wants some water now and again. He hasn't wanted a cigarette all day. For those who know him, this is unheard of. He's been a heavy smoker all his life. He says very little and it's often hard for him to say what he means. He hasn't had the energy to be out of bed for 3 days now and I know just lying down is becoming painful. I'm assuming his body wants to stretch and move... and he's too weak, with too little energy. His skin is tender to the touch, so we have to be careful touching him or moving him in the bed.

My wish for a magic wand is sooooo strong right now. And there isn't one. I can sit with him, but he's the only one who can allow peace and grace for himself. My heart aches so much it hurts. All I know to do is surround him with love.

A personal challenge has been dealing with a mother / daughter caretaker team who stole some of John's morphine. This was discovered by the Hospice nurse on Monday when she did her weekly check. A number of things/behaviors clicked at that point. I've reported it to the State Police. I'm now learning this duo has been pulling the wool over other people's eyes as well.

I have, however, found another caretaking team. These folks are on the Hospice caretaker list and many Hospice workers have hired them when their own family members needed assistance.

His oldest son visited today, very tearful. He told John, many times, tenderly, "I love you." I left them alone for the most part but I did see John holding his son's hands tightly. It was very good.

Your prayers and love are holding me up and together. Thank you

* * *

The hospice nurse said John has hours to days left. That was about 11 hours ago. He's still here. Cancer is so cruel. He's being eaten alive from the inside.

I'm past exhausted.

We both need your prayers and love so much right now. Thank you.

Thursday, September 19, 2019

Elmdea, to John's group:

John is still with us and is very peaceful now. He's not in pain, breathing easily. He's unresponsive, but I know he can hear. There have been many instances of divine orchestration today. Many.

His youngest son came to say his goodbyes this evening. I could only hear their voices and the tones, not the words. It sounded like he was pouring his heart out to his father. Such love was spoken and given. There is beauty all around.

Thursday, September 19, 2019

(near noon)

I've had an awareness. When John was switched to liquid meds (he was having trouble swallowing pills), I'd noticed that, while his breathing was fine, there was a kind of muscle fluttering in his abdomen. That scared me, so I began giving him his pain med every six hours instead of every four. It's back to every four hours. I'm really hoping I didn't increase his pain by going to six hours twice today.

I've realized in the past few days that I've been projecting how I imagined I'd feel in the same situation. Problem with that is: there's no way I could or can know how he's feeling, physically or emotionally. I'm still not explaining this very clearly.

I know John doesn't want to feel pain. I also know he doesn't want to be muzzy headed from the pain meds. But, at this point in his body's process, that's no longer possible. It's one more step on this awful journey he's on. But for him to be in pain and anxious just doesn't work now, for either of us.

Another part of my resistance was the fear that, at dying, his spirit/soul would be too confused to be able to leave and move on to the joy and beauty that awaits.

My fear that the opiates would interfere with John's passing is actually an indicator of my exhaustion. What I know (and had forgotten) is that the drugs, by diminishing pain and anxiety, allow the soul an easier exit, unimpeded by the anxieties of the mind and pains of the body.

But now, the definition of "comfort" is about keeping John seriously sedated and pain free.

As for me, I'm deeply exhausted in a way I've never been before. I'm not driving right now. I'm not alert enough. I got some decent sleep last night, thanks to a fan running in the bedroom so my mind couldn't stay alert for sounds from downstairs.

It's also helping that the new caregiver team is on board and I can relax about his care. They are also making sure I'm OK.

Thursday, September 19, 2019

Elmdea, to John's group:

> John is still with us. He hasn't had any water for about a day and a half now.

> I'm grateful beyond any words I have for a number of you (you know who you are) who will be sure his spirit doesn't get stuck after he exits this body.

> I have sensed the spirits of his departed family here, in great and tender love.

Friday, September 20, 2019

Another migraine. It woke me up around 6, later than usual. I went downstairs for my CBD tincture. On my way back upstairs, I stopped by John's bed.

"Another migraine, sweetie. I'll be ok." I touched his shoulder, then went back upstairs. Linda, the nighttime caregiver, just watched quietly. She is a comforting presence. I am beyond grateful for her care of both of us.

Sometime in that between awake and asleep space, I saw John sit up and swing his legs around to the floor. He was fully dressed in his jeans, t-shirt, red flannel shirt, and worn-out tennies; no catheter; no liver spots on his hands; no shingles on his head. He stood up, easily, and began walking toward the front hall.

In my dream, I thought "Oh no! What if he comes upstairs and sees I've cleaned off the top of his dresser. He'll be so upset."

And he was gone.

Not long after, I heard Linda call, "Elmdea! Come down. Now!"

I bolted up in bed. I bent over, shaking, as I fumbled my feet into my slippers. "This must be it. I have to be there. No, it can't be. It is." I stood, grabbed my bathrobe, and pulled it on as I went down the stairs.

Linda was waiting for me there. She touched my arm, lightly and compassionately. "Remember. He will still be able to hear you up to four minutes after he takes his last breath."

I nodded. "Thank you for reminding me."

I reached his bedside and lay my hand over his. Linda brought in a chair from the kitchen and left the living room. I sat so I could look straight at him. His breathing was a little erratic.

"I love you, John. I'm going to miss you… a lot. And I'll be OK."

My thoughts and my heart didn't agree. I wasn't at all sure I'd be OK. His breathing was still changing. I held his hand, silent, waiting for his next breath.

"I love you."

Then he took another breath, a pause. And another, a longer pause. A shallower breath. I waited for the next one. It never came. I realized I didn't know if that last breath was in or out. Not that it mattered. There wasn't one. His chest hadn't moved at all with that last breath. I didn't know if his last breath had been in or out. It was strange. How could I not know?

In my next breath, I felt disbelief, acceptance, completion, and sorrow settle in. He was gone. His life was done.

Unplanned and unwished for, my life with him was over. He was free. Free from the pain, the mental confusion and dullness from the meds, the helplessness in the face of cancer's greed. He was gone, irretrievably gone.

I knew it would happen and I wasn't ready.

His life was complete. Mine was not.

A feeling of finality.

"This is it."

I continued to sit by him, holding his hand, caressing his face, his beard. Talking to him.

"We've done this life dance many times before and we'll do it many times again."

I suspect I was talking more to myself than to him, attempting to forestall my own grief, my own knowing that never again will I see him breath, get a hug, a wry grin, a dissertation on something, a wild story that makes me laugh, the love and gentleness that were his hallmark, the messiness, the wobbling piles of papers and books...

I cupped his face, feeling the roughness of his beard. His beard, that had grown back a little curly after he lost it all to chemo.

"I love you. I love you so much."

Tears welled up.

His mouth was sagging open. I tried to close it. I really wanted it closed. It really wasn't going to. No matter.

I stood and bent over him, kissed his forehead, stroked his face some more, knowing these would be the last few times I could do this. It was so strange, this stillness. John truly had left his body. There was absolutely no energy there, just total limpness and stillness. An absence of John.

I remembered a friend commenting on feeling the life energy leave her husband's body when he died. That didn't happen with John. I didn't feel anything. He'd left it earlier, when I'd seen him get up. His poor cancer-ravaged body was just catching up.

It was sometime after 8. My mind decided on 8:12. I don't know why.

I sat with him a few minutes longer and the daytime caregiver arrived, a little late, thankfully.

First, I called Suwaylu. She said she'd come right away. Then I messaged his kids, as they'd requested. Then I texted Mara, so she could tell his dad. I'd thought it all out beforehand. There was no way I wanted anyone close hearing about John's death on social media.

Somewhere in there, I called Hospice, because they needed to come out, confirm his death, and fill out the death certificate. One of the additional blessings of hospice is that, when a person dies in their care, there's no need for an autopsy, which can take days. I assume that's the same in all states, but maybe not. It's true in West Virginia.

Linda came in and said they would get him cleaned up and dressed and I needed to go get his clothes. I went upstairs. Standing in front of his dresser, I still didn't believe it was real. I shook myself and opened his t-shirt drawer. Yes, this one. It was worn out, much loved. It had a large sun on it, the logo of a festival John went to before we met. What else? Oh, socks, some jeans, I guess he doesn't really need underwear. That was in another drawer. Oh, a flannel shirt, part of his uniform. His shoes, the old sneakers, with the toe starting to shred. They were the most comfortable and he kept wearing them, even though he had new ones, same style, just not broken in yet. Holding them all in my arms, I went downstairs.

Linda was just finishing washing him up. He was on his side, his bare ass white and small. Together, we got the t-shirt and shirt on, the jeans. The shoes and socks were easy. I made sure his scrimshawed Bridget medallion was centered on his chest, his hands crossed over his lower stomach. And his mouth was still open. I now understood why, in times past, there would often be a bandana tied under the jaw over the head: to keep the mouth closed. I just didn't have it in me to do that.

Then my sister called, asking why I'd called. Except... I hadn't called her yet. I didn't have my phone on me, so it wasn't a butt call. We both suspect John had something to do with that.

When Suwaylu arrived, she said an osprey (which was John's favorite bird) had swooped down next to her car as she was leaving her house. She could hear John saying "Tell her the old bird is free. The old bird is free!" and then the osprey flew off. Osprey aren't common around here.

The hospice nurse arrived and confirmed that John was dead and called the crematory to come pick up his body. John's oldest son had also arrived. We all just sat and waited, sometimes crying, sometimes not.

When the crematory van arrived, they came in with their stretcher. I told them they could take the sheet and pillow that John was on, so they did. I asked them not to cover his face, to wait until he was in the van. They did.

So John got to leave his home, facing the sky, carried down the front steps. When he first came to look at this house, he'd walked around outside and found a peach tree with ripe peaches on it. He grabbed one and was eating it, sitting on the front steps, when the realtor arrived. "I'm buying this house," he said. "Don't you need to see inside?" she asked. "No. This is my house." And it was.

It was good his oldest son was there. As John was taken down the steps, the wheeled stretcher almost collapsed. His son caught it, keeping his father from rolling off onto the ground.

The stretcher was rolled into the van, the van doors closed, and they drove away. I watched the van until it disappeared around a corner. John is gone. Forever gone. A loud wailing keen rose from deep within as I watched that van disappear, carrying John away from me forever.

The pain. Like no pain I've ever known. He's gone.

Friday, September 20, 2019

(Elmdea to both groups)

John died peacefully this morning. I was holding his hand as he took his last breaths. His spirit had left his body sometime earlier, his body was just catching up with that reality. He's free.

* * *

A friend posted this on John's page:

"What is remembered, lives. Hail the goer.
Nine nights from tonight, I will go to the graveyard next to our
building and pray this final prayer to his spirit:
I release you beloved
from any constraint on you I may have
My arms no longer hold you.
My fingers loose their grasp
My eyes do not look on you
My lips do not speak your name to bid you stay.
Thus freed, the choice is yours, to go or linger to bless,
or join the mighty ones who went before us all."

* * *

Another friend posted this:

"In the night of death, hope sees a star, and listening love can hear the
rustle of a wing."

Looking Back

John rallied from late July through early August. That's a term frequently used by Hospice and those writing about this process: the dying will have a brief rally of awareness and mobility before they die. The sources I read said it was usually in the days or hours before death. That didn't happen with John. His rally was two months before he died. Yet another example of how each death is unique.

Hospice provided weekly nurses visits, emotional and spiritual counseling, medication management and delivery, and 24/7 phone availability. I had thought Hospice (in general) offered caregiving, too. It turns out very few do.

I'm soooo grateful I was able to keep my promises to John: that he would die at home and I would be with him when he died. I later realized he was terrified of hospitals. I'll never know why.

"Seeing" John sit up and calmly walk away from his bed in his signature outfit of jeans, t-shirt, and a flannel shirt was such a gift. That "seeing" let me know he was ready and had fully exited his body. My psychopomp friends later confirmed that they knew when his soul departed and that it was an easy passage, requiring no assistance from them. The Hospice Chaplain was right: John had found grace. May we all be so blessed.

PART VIII: WIDOWHOOD

Sunday, September 22, 2019

It's been 2 days since John's death. My emotions are up and down, all over the place. Yesterday I was so grief-stricken I wanted to die. It didn't help that I've been having cluster migraines. Last night and part of this morning, I felt fairly normal. I know these swings and the places between are my new normal for awhile. I'm actively practicing not holding on to the times of respite and remembering that the deep grief isn't forever.

I still need all of you. I'll still be posting here. This space allows me to process and be witnessed.

Sunday, September 22, 2019

Elmdea, to John's group:

I thank you and John's spirit thanks you for your love, your support, and your rituals and healings during this journey. I won't be making many more posts here. I have a similar group to this I set up for my support, as John set this one up for his. Many of you are in both groups. If you would like me to send you an invitation to my group, please message me.

Monday, September 23, 2019

John's obituary
(shared in both groups; edited to protect privacy)

John P. Adams, Jr. of Berkeley Springs, WV, died peacefully at home on September 20, 2019, after a long and painful journey with cancer. He was born February 16, 1950, the son of

** and **. He is survived by his father; his wife, his three children; and two grandchildren.

John served as the Prosecuting Attorney for Morgan County in the 1990's. He went on to serve as a Public Defender in the Martinsburg office, retiring in 2012. His proudest moment was arguing a case before the West Virginia Supreme Court and receiving a compliment from one of the judges for the quality of his brief.

John began drinking at a young age. By the time he was 29, he knew alcohol would kill him before he was 30 unless he quit. He went into residential treatment, followed by many years of active membership in AA. At the time of his death, he had completed 40 years of sobriety. He was able to do this because he was willing to look at the good and the dark sides of himself, working with them, doing what he could to resolve them. This, in turn, made him a man of great compassion, understanding, and wisdom, although he would claim none of those for himself.

At his death, he was a respected and beloved elder in his local and spiritual communities. Friends describe him as a man of quick wit, with a loving heart, a wry smile, and a wicked sense of humor, a gifted storyteller, a man of his word, a great listener, and a mentor. He would often be reading five books at once ranging from history to science fiction to philosophy. He loved MMO's and interacting with guild members. He deep sea dove to wrecks off the southern US coast. He had an abiding love of cats. He loved his wife's pot roast. He hoped he would be remembered as someone who tried and did some different things in his life, who was intelligent and curious, and who was a good friend. His hopes are fulfilled.

This poem was cherished by John, posted in his meditation and prayer area.

The limbs that move, the eyes that see,
These are not entirely me;
Dead men and women helped to shape,
The mold that I do not escape;
The words I speak, the written line,
These are not uniquely mine.
For in my heart and in my will,
Old ancestors are warring still,
Celt, Roman, Saxon and all the dead,
From whose rich blood my veins are fed,
In aspect, gesture, voices, tone,
Flesh of my flesh, bone of my bone;
In fields they tilled, I plow the sod,
I walk the mountain paths they trod;
Around my daily steps arise—
The good, the bad – those I comprise.
          – Richard Rolle 1300 – 1349

Tuesday, September 24, 2019

I had an awareness last night. I need to run some errands in town today, including dropping off John's shower transfer bench, walker, and a number of other things at the Senior Center. Joyce will be helping me load them in my car early this afternoon. My mind automatically went to "I'll run the other errands then, cuz Joyce will be here."

Then it hit me. I don't need to make sure anyone is here at home. I don't need to have a worry in the back of my mind about how John is doing. Oh. I hadn't realized how embedded that was until now, when it doesn't need to be anymore.

I don't think it's really sunk home yet how truly gone his physical presence is.

Tuesday, September 24, 2019

Elmdea, to both groups:

As I requested, the crematory just called to let me know that John's body will be going into the crematory in the next five minutes, so around 11:50 this morning, eastern time. In about 2-3 hours, his body will be ashes. I'm energetically standing with him as his body enters Bridget's forge and fire. Holding space for me and for him now.

I also asked for his weight. He weighed 179 pounds, only 4 less than it did near the end of June. But he was so much more gaunt.

Most of his ashes will be in a large urn and will go home with his father. John was his only child. It only seems right. I have a number of mini urns that the Crematory will put some of his ashes in, some for his kids, some for me.

Thursday, September 26, 2019

My sister arrived from Arizona yesterday and she'll be here for 2 weeks. I'm grateful.

Joyce has spent every night here since John died so I wouldn't be sleeping in an empty house. Thank you soooo much, Joyce!

I'm learning the landscape of grief after death. It is, indeed, different from anticipatory grief. It rises more often, more freely. I suspect part of that is I no longer feel the need (or have the need) to keep it under control so I'm not in meltdown if John needs me.

I've discovered two things (so far), going through his things. I'm still learning new things about him. It's part of what I treasured about our relationship. The other is that what I most need to get rid of now are the bits and pieces directly related to this last 9 or so months, as the cancer began and sped up its consumption of his body.

In going through pictures for his memorial, I've realized the cancer began sapping his energy 3-4 years ago. It was very gradual, because esophageal cancer is a slow growing cancer with very few symptoms until it's near or has reached Stage 4, when it's impossible to reverse.

Friday, September 27, 2019

My sister and I picked up John's ashes today. When we got home, it felt like John had come home.

A few days ago, I found a small box amongst John's things. It now holds his still running watch, his wedding ring, and some other small things that represent events and people important to him. I've set that box, along with a small blue urn of his ashes (blue was his favorite color) and some flowers on a small table. A small altar.

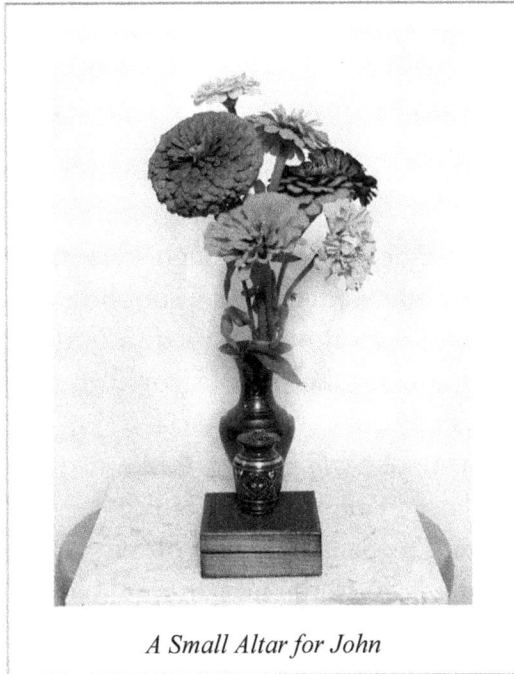

A Small Altar for John

Welcome home, my love. I know your spirit is near and I'm grateful. I know you'll be traveling on at some point and these small things carry the imprint of you. Thank you.

Saturday, September 28, 2019

We had the family gathering and wake today. It went well. It was good to meet some of John's family members I'd only heard him speak of. I'd asked the Hospice Chaplain to come so he could share what he could about John. We talked some during the meal. I said I didn't much like being a widow. He said widow was an honorable title. It meant I'd honored my commitment of "'til death do us part." That's true. And I don't like being a widow.

I remember what the Druid priestess said at our handfasting: that John and I are "bound together, through this life and those following, whether you stay together in this life or not." John has left this life. I find comfort that we'll be together again at some point.

Sunday, September 29, 2019

It's been over a week now and it still doesn't seem real that John's gone.

Becky and I have been going through some things. Sometimes it's easy and sometimes it's sooooo not.

Today, the librarian from the Morgan County Public Library came out to see if any of John's books could go on their shelves. There were frequent little squeals of joy. He would be happy to know his books will be read by many others. She said they'd get bookplates made for them, indicating they're gifts from John's estate. I'm glad some part of him gets to live on that way. The rest will go to the recycling center tomorrow, where patrons can adopt what they want.

I feel kind of groundless. The shape of my life has totally changed and I don't know where the new ground is, let alone what it looks or feels like.

Saturday, October 5, 2019

Today was the memorial service for John at the funeral home in town. A good number of John's friends and his co-workers from the public defender's office attended. When Suwaylu played *Amazing Grace*, I cried. John did find grace. I'm so grateful he did.

Several people mentioned they "saw" John there and he was nodding his head in approval at the proceedings.

Monday, October 7, 2019

My new (smaller) Roku TV arrived today and I've installed Prime on it. The old, great big one that John loved to watch football on went to the Chapel.

Thursday, October 10, 2019

My sister left for home today. I'm grateful she was able to come out for two weeks. It's made this time easier. Tonight will be my first night alone in the house since John died. I'm ready for some alone time. I think I need it, to begin settling into what my life is now.

Monday, October 14, 2019

Going through John's stuff is strange. We so respected each other's things and spaces and now? As I go through the secretary in the living room, I'm finding bits of this and that, pictures, notes, medallions, cards. I've no idea what they meant to him. They meant something because many of them (pictures, notes) are from years ago.

I've no words for the emptiness of that. They are literally just "stuff". A life gone, the memories gone, absent, no more. Leaving everything as he'd left it doesn't change that. John's not here to care or remember. Where he is, his things are just that: things.

Wednesday, October 19, 2019

Today I sorted through John's clothes. Ties, sport coats, jeans, t-shirts, fleece vests, cloaks, tunics, leather motorcycle vest, shoes, all of it. I've sorted the cloaks, tunics, and leather gear into one pile, which I'll take to a gathering of close friends at the end of this month. Most of his t-shirts and flannel shirts are going into a rolling duffle, for me. I might turn them into a rag rug, or memory bears or I dunno. I just don't want to let them go.

Then there's the big pile. He used to shop at Goodwill (he so loved finding bargains) and said it was always hard to find things in his size (XXXL and Size 13½ shoe). For starters, it seems men wear stuff out so there isn't necessarily much that's worth going to Goodwill or Salvation Army.

Wednesday, October 23, 2019

Today, I took the big pile of John's clothes and shoes to the Rescue Mission here in town. It's a way he can give back to this community that he loved and lived in for thirty years.

I was OK, loading the car. It took a few trips around the block to find the Rescue Mission. It wasn't open, but there was a shed with a note on it. It said "Donations Can Be Left Here." So I did.

Driving home, I almost had to pull over I was crying so hard. One more piece of him gone. But keeping all those clothes wouldn't bring him back. Nothing will. Nothing. I miss him so much. Words can't come close.

Wednesday, November 6, 2019

I've been wishing for almost a week now that the weather would get really awful so I could cancel my trip out west. I know I need to see my mother and I'm afraid to leave home. I'm afraid that, if I leave, I'll lose John. That staying here will help keep some part of him here with me.

I know it doesn't make any logical sense.

The weather isn't cooperating, so Anne will drop me off in Hancock in the morning so I can catch the shuttle to BWI.

But I'm leaving John, somehow.

Wednesday, November 13, 2019

I flew back today. I took the shuttle to Frederick, where Joyce picked me up. That felt strange. It's always been John before. Now it isn't. And won't ever be again.

I'm home. My grief is present. John's absence is present. I haven't lost John. I've lost some of the craziness, at least for now.

The trip was hard. Neither my mother or sister really understand my grief. They've never experienced this kind of deep grief. Yes, they've lost people, but I'm understanding they weren't as close to them as I was to John, so their grief was different. I just hurt. Lots. And then I don't for a few minutes. Then I do again. I think I'm doing pretty well, until I look back and review and realize, no, I'm managing. I'm not doing well. There's a difference.

Thursday, December 5, 2019

Elmdea: This new path without John is difficult. I hadn't ever envisioned the future without him.

Mel: Indeed it is Elmdea. Bless you, friend. I know how difficult it truly is. I'm praying for you and sending big love and warm hugs during the holidays and each step of your way. Reach out anytime Elmdea.

Kit: It's the hardest thing for anyone to go through....hugs!

Paula: I know exactly how you feel. It is difficult. However we somehow go on to create a new life for ourselves. Sending love and hugs.

Deb: We understand. Tell us about one of your favorite memories, if you would like.

Elmdea: John had a way of spinning and telling stories that got me laughing almost every time.

Bev: the best storyteller.

Elmdea: so much the best. And he never really wrote them down

Bev: you can write them down.

Elmdea: Some I could. Others? They were spur of the moment. He was so masterful at those. Got me laughing soooo many times. I had to watch him cuz sometimes they were about something that actually happened, others times not so much, as in created in that moment. His face would give him away at some point with the imaginary stories. He was gooooood at those.

Nel: When my father was dying he had been sedated and could hear but not move or speak. I realized later I was given the opportunity to learn how to communicate when he was no longer present physically. I'm not meaning spirit – just learning to listen for the presence that is always there, in your thinking, and your memories, like a listening for your speaking where you "feel" or "sense" the response. I understood it to be like an energy signature. I don't know if this helps but I felt it right to mention it here.

Elmdea: Thank you. What you shared is a confirmation of something that I've been aware of. I've touched on who/what he is now: his essence is vast. Who he was here is a very small part of that vastness and I still sense that, too, now and again.

Sal – and its winter and its cold and you can't really go outside much and work off any sadness etc, and the holidays where it seems like most folks have family around – all that does not help – I know you must feel lonely and lost, this is always the hardest time, when the funeral and trips and visits end and then you are alone. I'm so sorry.

Jenna – Blessings on your journey ~ one day at a time ~ feel your feelings and grieve hard! Loss isn't easy ~ I know… my husband died when I was 30…

Julie – Establishing a new normal is hard, just hard. Sometimes simply admitting that can help.

Cat: Facing the future minus the love of your life has got to be unimaginably hard. It's just not supposed to happen this way. Your lives together had just begun and were so rich with promise.

I'd like to find the god/goddess/spirit responsible for this terrible plan. I have some thoughts I'd like to share.

I know you are surrounded by a loving community, and am so grateful on your behalf for that. And I know nothing and no one will take John's place in that empty space he's left behind.

Elmdea: It's the promise of what we now can't share. As for Who to speak to about this, it was his soul's journey, and therefore mine. It wasn't and isn't easy, but I wouldn't trade any of it. Knowing and being with him, though such a short time, was a gift I embrace.

Cat: Yes… it's that broken promise that is so hard to bear. You will forever embrace his gift

Marty: I am so sorry, hon. None of us expected that for you. You are welcome to come share the fire when I am around.

Wednesday, December 11, 2019

I just received something in the mail: a cute little red truck with surfboards in the back. The thing is: I've NO idea who it's from/where it came from. No gift tag, no return address.

And the little license plate # is HR1216. John's birthday was 2/16, he used to have a red truck, and he loved the ocean. Sooooo…

I know. A lot of synchronicities. I don't even collect things like this, but… questions, curiosity, gratitude…

I remember him saying a month or more before my birthday that he had taken care of getting me something. This might be it, just very delayed. I'm considering it a gift from him.

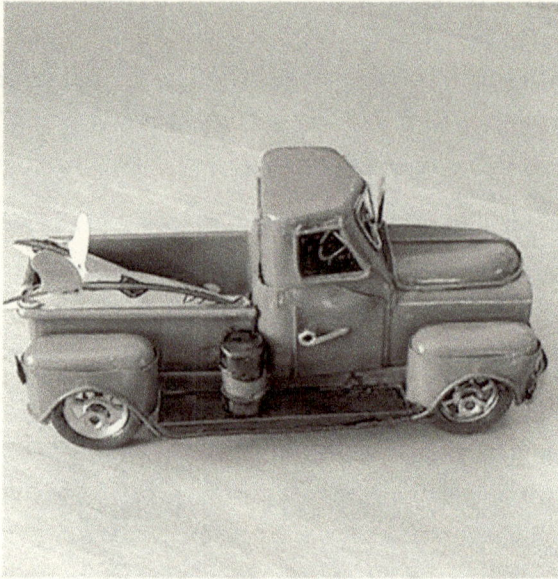

Surprise Red Truck, 2019

As one friend said:

"All signs point to someone who loves you. Enjoy your truck! You may never know the sender but I suspect, as one of your friends, John may have ordered it."

I wouldn't put it past him to do that. I mean… he called my sister from my phone about 45 minutes after he died. And it wasn't a butt call on my part.

Saturday, January 4, 2020

John Pavlovitz had a post about how bereaved people aren't strong, they're just trying to survive. It struck home for me and I commented on his post.

"My husband died 15 weeks ago after a year of being progressively ravaged by cancer and its treatments. I was his sole caregiver. I was aware of being broken open and shattered through all of it. Then, and still, people told me how strong I was. I didn't feel strong, I was doing the only thing I knew to do: love and care for him. I viewed (and continue to) that being broken open as his last gift to me, strange as that may sound. I vowed I wouldn't ignore or waste it. I'm deep in the continuing process of discovering who I am, as myself and as a person without her beloved. I'm unendingly grateful for my therapist; and for the grief counseling, groups, and memorial gatherings offered by Hospice. They've been and are a lifeline.

Some days are good, some not so much. I'm befriending my grief because it will always be with me, appearing when and as it will, often out of seemingly nowhere. Strong? Maybe. Mostly I think it's resilience because it's the only thing I know to do to honor his love and our love.

And yes, this blows."

I think it was back in June, about when John entered Hospice care, when I wrote that I thought my grief for John would be somewhat like my grief for my cats: intense for a bit, then dwindling. I had no idea how wrong I was. No idea. I thought anticipatory grief was just like after death grief.

It's not.

Anticipatory grief just scratches the surface of the deep, soul-wrenching, life-changing death of a beloved.

Monday, February 10, 2020

My new propane tank was delivered today! Now I don't have to worry about running out of fuel if the power goes out for a week or more. My electrician helped me figure out what would work best. I now have a large generator that's wired to the furnace, appliances and kitchen/office. All I have to do is switch the electricity to the generator breakers, crack the 3rd "porch" door open, start the fan, and start the generator. No pull starts. No long lengths of electrical cord to run all over the house, like John and I used to do. I've test started the generator and it works perfectly. I'm beyond relieved.

Wednesday, February 12, 2020

I've been meaning to write about my week at Superstars, the writing conference I was at last week. However, grief has raised its head again. There are five things coming up.

First: the 15th – the one year anniversary of when we found out John had Stage 4 cancer and he decided to go for chemo.

Second: the 16th – John's 70th birthday.

Third: the 19th – a colonoscopy/endoscopy. I'm due, I don't like them, but I'll absolutely go get one. Joyce is taking me up there (Hagerstown) and then spending the night after here, cuz the anesthetic messes with my brain and I'm loopy for a few days, worst on the day of. I'd asked John to get one several times over the last few years of his life. He refused. If he had, he might still be alive. So many ifs.

Fourth: the 20th – 5 months since John's death. It seems like forever ago and no time at all.

Fifth: I have what I hope is only a cold, so my energy is low, I'm tired, etc.

I saw my grief counselor on Tuesday. She said that, often, the lead ups to significant anniversaries are harder than the anniversaries themselves. Time will tell.

* * *

Topic change.

I met with an agent at Superstars. She's very interested in the caretaking book and suggested I fictionalize it, since autofic is big right now. Autofic is "autobiographical fiction," which I hadn't heard of before. Who knew? I told her it would be 1-2 years before I could get it to her. She was good with that.

I also went to something called "The Eggs Benedict Breakfast." It's hosted by James A. Owen who has written a number of books, including the *Meditations Trilogy*. At the end of it, he had these small cards, about 1" x 3", each with a quote from these books. He fanned them out in his hand, the backs of the cards facing each of us as he walked around the table. The one that called to me and that I drew broke me open.

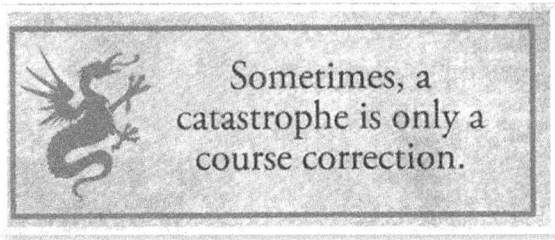

Sometimes, a catastrophe is only a course correction.

After I got home, LeAnne posted something similar:

"Not all storms come to disrupt your life. Some come to clear your path."

To me, they say pretty much the same thing: John's death was a catastrophic storm in my life. I've no real idea what my path forward is other than taking things a step at a time. I'm still finding my way, and it's a twisted path, rather than the nice straight logical one I'd like.

Those of you who've known me for many years know I can withdraw into my head. I'd been doing that. That card put me solidly back in my heart, and my grief. I'm missing John a great deal, some of it wistful, some painful, tears arising very easily. What I'm remembering more are the years we had together and small incidents, conversations, life stuff, rather than the horror and anguish of the last 7 months of his life. In the long run, that's a good thing, even though it doesn't feel so great right now.

Thursday, February 13, 2020

Update: The colonoscopy/endoscopy has been rescheduled for April 15. Why? Cuz I woke up with tonsillitis this morning and they won't do anesthesia for 2 weeks after upper respiratory anything. Too risky. The soonest was April 1 or 15. So NOT doing it on April Fools, lol.

I'm grateful I still have my tonsils and they're doing their job. Called Dr. Grant and I'll have antibiotics soon.

Friday, February 14, 2020

I got a private message from a woman who'd known John since they were in college. It reassured me in a way I needed, to know I'd made that much difference to John and his life.

Bev: Happy valentines. I believe you were the love of John's life. 🖤 *no stress, no over analyzing, no peer pressure. Just pure love. Have a peaceful day.*

Elmdea: Thank you. We felt very blessed to have found each other. He was the love of my life too. I miss him soooooooooooooo much.

Bev: It did not go unnoticed by me and other of my University friends who do not comment. With you he shared peace of mind. That was a missing link for most of his life. You gave that to him.

Elmdea: Thank you, deeply. I had sensed that but couldn't know, since I didn't know him before. I'm grateful I could provide that for him, as he did for me. I know he wants me to grieve and re-engage with life. But it's hard without him. I will, to honor him and his memory.

Bev: May the force be with you. I feel strongly that you deserve support for your dignity and total awareness that only you could have experienced with John as a fully formed being. My love to you

🖤🖤

Sunday, February 16, 2020

This will be a longish post, but I promise it'll be worth it. For those of you in both my group and John's, it's the same post.

This past week was really hard, with two anniversaries coming up: meeting with the medical oncologist on the 15th and learning that John definitely had Stage 3, possibly Stage 4, cancer and John immediately opting for chemo; and today, the 16th, being John's 70th birthday. I spent a lot of time in tears this past week, talking to John, crying some more. Friday evening, Suwaylu called and offered to bring me lunch and help me glue together the toy Viking ship I'll use to send some of John's ashes to the ocean. I'd had other plans yesterday, but my intuition said this was important.

Suwaylu and I were sitting on the couch and I was sharing how John hated having a February birthday because it's cold and dark. When he could, he'd go on a Caribbean cruise.

Then John came through to Suwaylu (she's been able to hear messages from the other side for most of her life) and he said for me to remember where and how he's celebrating now. I looked up and had a *huge* ah-hah moment! He's on the absolutely ultimate cruise in an ocean of total unconditional love.

Suwaylu and I talked a little about the blocks to love. I do my best, as did John, as does Suwaylu , as we all do – and we're all human with blocks to giving and receiving love. It's part of this human experience. And John's now entirely free of those blocks. He's MORE than fine!

Then John was right between us (I could sense him) and he bent down and said to Suwaylu "She's a little slow sometimes." Suwaylu shared that and I immediately, without even thinking about it, turned and flipped him off. Why? Because that comment was and is *so* John. I could "hear" him saying that. He used to tell me things and sometimes, they were totally made up and I didn't "get it" until he broke out laughing, at which point, yeah, I'd sometimes flip him off, ruefully laughing at myself.

Yesterday, John roared with laughter after I flipped him off and we joined in. I could energetically sense his laughter. It was beyond wonderful. For Suwaylu and me, it was full-bodied laughter, like neither of us have had for quite a while. It was wonderful! When the laughter subsided, we were both aware that our blocks to love's awareness had cleared.

At which point, John said "and that's the laughing staff." He was referring to the staff he'd created before we met, using wand lore and ritual, lunar cycles, water, sandpaper (lots of sandpaper). It's absolutely imbued with his energy… and it's unfinished. Since he died, I've been looking at it, collecting stones and sparkly things, considering, wanting to honor him and his work.

Soooo, since John declared it the laughing staff – I got out the amethyst sphere and, with Suwaylu's help, I super glued it to the top of the staff. There wasn't any (self-imposed) need any more to be ritually careful with how I finished it or decorated it. It's time to just love it, have fun, and play as I finish it. It may never be finished, but I will be using it.

I feel lighter today. John wanted to be on a cruise to celebrate his 70th birthday. He is. Not quite the way he'd envisioned it a year ago… and it's far more beautiful and wonderful than any earthly cruise. Please join me in celebrating John's birthday wish come true.

FYI – the Viking ship still isn't glued together, lol. It will be.

* * *

Some of his friends sent him birthday messages in his group page:

- *Remembering you fondly, my dear friend. Happy birthday in the great beyond! Miss you.*
- *Forever in our hearts as we remember you fondly today. 70… hope you are celebrating your best life, wherever you may be on your journey.*
- *Remembering…*
- *Grateful I had the privilege of knowing you, John. May your journey and birthday be blessed.*
- *Thinking of you today with much gratitude and love.*
- *I wish you well and happy in the world beyond, where all is bright and there is no pain and strife. Happy birthday, John, your memory is not gone.*

Looking Back

At the time, I thought I was functioning as I had before this all started. I believed I was handling everything really well. I wasn't. For instance, I forgot to put checks and debit card purchases in my check register and monitor my balance, so I got overdrawn a few times. That was new and very unlike the old me, prior to John's death.

I realize now that I was doing what most people do after such a deep loss. I had grief brain, a very real thing. My memory was faulty, I had a short attention span, and decisions felt overwhelming. I fell back on old patterns and wondered who I actually was. My grief was intense. My world had fundamentally changed. I had no idea how I fit into it or who I really was anymore.

I didn't mention it in my posts or my journal, but I remember counting the hours, then the days, then the weeks since John had died. Then the months and weeks. Then the months. I was still trying to wrap my head and my heart around his physical absence. I even figured out the date at which I would have lived longer than John. It seemed important at the time. I wrote it in my calendar to make sure I'd remember.

I kept checking John's watch to see if it had stopped. As of this writing it was still running, but had lost about six hours. Why don't I just pull out the watch stem to stop it? Because it feels like a tenuous connection to John when he was alive. The paradoxes of grief: I could let go of 99% of his clothes in the first few weeks after his death but I can't stop his watch, it has to stop on its own.

Western culture considers six months long enough to grieve before we need to leave it all behind and get on with life. Deep grief doesn't work that way. But we grievers do our best to hide it. Everyone around us has moved on with their lives. We are stumbling forward in our radically changed world. We aren't *moving on* because we can't and won't leave that part of our life behind. We *move forward*, step by step, carrying our grief and our love, trying to find our way in a world that we recognize yet which is also utterly alien.

I made plans to do some Road Scholar trips that would take me away from home for a week or so. Joyce said she'd look in on Alice for me. I thought I was re-engaging with life. But life had other plans for all of us.

Part IX:
The Pandemic Arrives

Monday, March 16, 2020

Well… things have certainly changed in the world! I hope all of you are well.

As of today, I'm self-isolated. I'm well, feel great… and I want to stay that way. A few weeks ago, my intuition said to go get some food, some TP (lol), and some other supplies. I'm well stocked and there are some local younger folks who will run errands for me. While I'm concerned about Covid-19, I'm not in panic mode at all. I know it's going to get pretty intense in the next week or so and continue that way for a while. That said… I'd like to open this space up for all of you. You are part of my community. This is a safe space to share concerns, ideas, and we can support each other. I'm not viewing this space as "just for me" any more. It's now "for us."

From here on out, I'll be posting something here every 3 or 4 days. I'm alone in the house, except for Alice the cat. If I don't post, please give me a call. I'm asking this in case the solitude sends me into deep doldrums. I know the signs and plan to reach out before I go too far down the rabbit hole. I don't anticipate this will happen, me being an introvert and comfortable with my own company.

I'm also getting a Pro plan on Zoom so I can do virtual get-togethers with folks. Let me know if you'd like to do that, or FaceTime. I'm sooooo open to that.

Last week (Sunday morning) I woke up and looked out the window of my bedroom. There were the pine trees that John had so carefully mowed around for many years. I had them thinned a few weeks ago so the stronger ones could get even stronger. The memory brought me to tears. They were different tears though. The grief wasn't as sharp and tearing. They were also tears for…? And it was good.

Then I fell asleep again, mostly in that between sleep and awake state. While in that space, I found myself in the kitchen here at the house. I was making pancakes and there was also a bowl of melted chocolate. John and I were talking as I made the pancakes. "Why don't you dip the pancakes in the chocolate?" he said. So I did. They were pretty good. He liked them too. It was a most wonderful experience because it was soooooo ordinary, the way it was with John and me for most of our time together.

There are two other things that are wonderful about that "dream". First: I VERY rarely have people I know show up in my dreams. Second: this is the first time John has shown up in a dream and that we had a conversation.

Since then, I've felt more at peace. There are still tears, but the character of them has changed. They feel softer, less wrenching.

I've also started writing about our last year together. It is part of my healing. This Friday will mark 6 months since his death. It's now enough time that I can read over what I wrote here and in my journals, and not feel like I'm right back in it.

Since I'll be posting something here more often, I'll stop for now.

I love you all. Please stay well.

Tuesday, March 17, 2020

> *Deep within the still center of my being, may I find peace.*
> *Quietly in the circle of this grove, may I share peace.*
> *Gently within the circle of all life, may I radiate peace.*
> — Druid's Peace Prayer

Thank you, Dana, for reminding me of this.

Thursday, March 19, 2020

Medicare has approved something called "telehealth" so people can see their doctor without going to the office. The requirement is that it's both audio and visual, so FaceTime or ?

My BIG win for the day is… it also covers physical therapy! I had my first ever telehealth physical therapy session this morning. I'm so grateful and relieved. I had some minor but limiting issues come up and I now know how to work with them.

Friday, March 20, 2020

Today is six months since John died. I'm making peace with the fact he's no longer in body.

Tears still come and I welcome them. I no longer feel guilty if I haven't cried for several days. I seriously wish he was still here, but only if he could be fully healthy.

I'm pretty much self-isolating. The exception was getting stuff to my accountant. There are several people who will run errands for me if I need anything. I'm pretty well stocked, thanks to my intuitive Costco run a few weeks ago.

Sunday, March 22, 2020

I've had some near freak outs this week about self-isolation and Covid-19. I do my 4 square breathing, take a walk, consciously go do something. It helps.

I'm not sleeping all that well. I've realized it's familiar: it's how I slept when I was solo caretaking John, knowing I had no control over his cancer, much as I desperately wanted to. This is the same.

I'm picking up what helped me then: reading, weaving, writing, touching in with friends, and doing what's safely in reach to help or be of assistance to others, given I'm in self-isolation too and plan to stay that way.

I've started weaving my first set of towels on my mother's 30 year old rigid heddle loom. These towels are going to have lots of character since I'm learning and the edges aren't all that even. That's ok. I'm learning, having fun; and the colors, textures, and moving the shuttle back and forth are hugely soothing. I'll be weaving more rugs, cutting the strips, sewing them together, then playing with how the colors work together as I weave on the big rug loom, the loom John loved to hear me weaving on.

Saturday, April 4, 2020

I figured this would be happening at some point. Now it has. Governor Jim Justice has issued some tight restrictions for this part of the state because of the rise in Covid cases. I'm ok. I went to the bank (drive thru with the canister) today, first time I've left my property in 2 weeks. I wiped off my hands immediately afterwards with the Clorox wipes I brought with me.

In an unexpected way, the time I've grieved John, both before and after his death, is making this easier. I know the signs that my stress is ramping up and what I need to do to take care of me.

Wednesday, April 8, 2020

(from a friend)
> Cathi: *Hello dear Elmdea. Hope you're safe and feeling loved. We're all together in this*
> Elmdea: *Thank you, Cathi. I'm safe and I'm feeling loved, but I've had a few conversations with John about his timing. I'm grateful he left before this all happened and I sure wish he'd gotten on top of his health before it was too late cuz I'd sure like his company these days.*

Cathi: Yeah… a bit selfish of him don't ya think??? You can tell him that for me, please

Elmdea: I will. You can too. He'll probably get a chuckle out of it. Our conversations so far are totally one-sided.

Cathi: He'll laugh… I have no doubt! And yes… he "visits". We talk. But he's… 20? How does that happen?

Elmdea: cuz he gets to choose how he appears, and that's also how you knew him.

Cathi: And we had some unfinished business… which he appears to want to work out now. I hope it leaves him peaceful. I bear no grudges…

Elmdea: He was very focused on working out as many things as he could while he was living. I'm unsurprised he's continuing to do so.

Cathi: Interesting to know.

There was a conversation we really needed to have. But didn't. Always thought we'd get to it. But time ran out for him. I suppose he's circling back to tie those loose ends.

I've been hesitant to tell you this. But I suspect you know in some way. And it has no bearing on your relationship together. And… that he visits me now… it's somehow confusing and totally understandable at the same time.

Elmdea: I'm tickled to have this confirmation that he's alive and well on the other side.

He DID show up in a dream a month or so back and it was healing and beautiful in its ordinary-ness.

Cathi: Elmdea Oh yes… total confirmation that he is quite "alive" on the other side

Elmdea: You've sooooo made my day. Thank you.

Cathi: And he's got some 'splaining to do… .and is trying hard to come up with the answers he couldn't first go-round.

Elmdea: ROFLMAO!

Tuesday, April 14, 2020

I think I'm in week four of self-isolation. It's been up and down, emotionally. At this point, I'm in a place of calm, making peace with the fact that me staying home is the most important thing I can do.

I'm doing a bit more weaving. I've finished that towel and another one that's purple (no stripes) on my mother's old rigid heddle loom. For a first try, they're coming out pretty well.

I continue to enjoy (and really, really need, for sanity and exercise) my daily walks, including discovering that Sassafras trees have blossoms!.

Like many others, I've tried my hand at baking. I made Brown Irish Soda Bread. It's pretty tasty and lasts well in the fridge.

Wednesday, April 15, 2020

With everything else going on, I lost track of the release date of the anthology, *X Marks the Spot*. (I mean, there were, what, 348 days in March and 127 so far in April?) I know a great many of the authors and I'm honored to be in their company. There are ghost stories, sci fi, fantasy, and mystery, just to name a few genres.

My story, *Life Pirate*, is about a clump of cancer cells. I wrote it while I was care-giving John. It will be added at the end of this book. I've realized it's part of it.

Monday, April 20, 2020

Now my county is in official lockdown. Sigh. It's going to be a long spring, summer, and winter. John and I had talked about something like this happening, but we figured we'd be together. While I love Miz Alice, she's a cat. There's only so much she can do.

The other thing that's happened is that the three Road Scholar weeks I'd signed up for have also been cancelled. I was really looking forward to them. So many things being put on hold.

And I have grief brain. I know I thought I was handling things well last October. Then a few months later, looking back, I realize I was so-so. That is still happening. Grief is a strange creature.

The pandemic has ensured that I'll be staying in the house for at least a year. At this point, I'm not even sure I'm ready to leave the memories. The place in the kitchen where we stood when, unbeknownst to me, we had our last husband / wife hug, rather than caretaker / invalid hugs. His place at the kitchen table. His bed and how he'd prop himself up to read, munching on something. His office chair, where he'd play RPG for hours. His chair on the front porch, where we had so many wonderful conversations.

So many memories. I'm not ready to let them go.

Friday, May 15, 2020

Nine years ago today, John and I were handfasted by a Druid Priestess at Blue Ridge Beltane. It was a beautiful and special ritual and heart-joining.

Every year after, John and I would go outside, then take 5 steps away from each other. At that point, we could continue walking and leave, no harm no foul, or we could turn back to each other. Every year, we turned back to each other, committing ourselves to each other for another year.

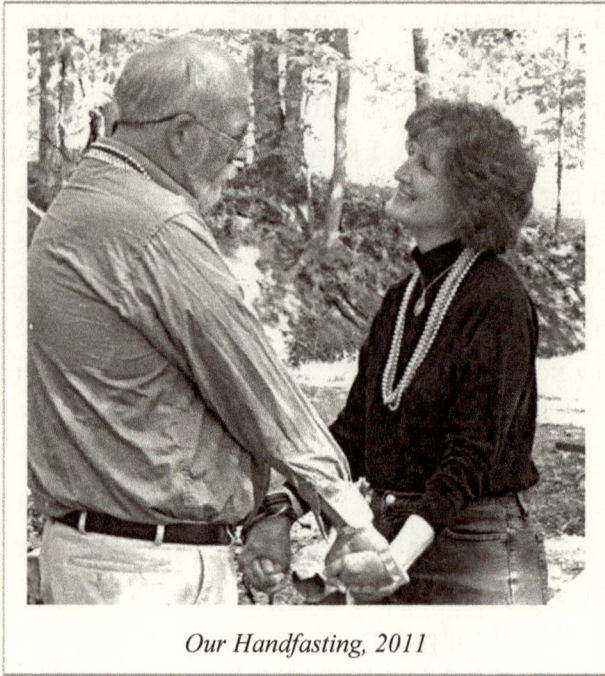

Our Handfasting, 2011

Last year, John was in a small room at the Marsh Cancer Center in Hagerstown, getting IV saline after a radiation treatment. I told him it was the 8th anniversary of our handfasting and I would walk to the door and he could either open his eyes to say he was staying, or close them to say he was leaving. I turned back to him and his eyes were wide open.

This year... he's still here, in his own way. This morning, I opened the freezer door to get out the blueberries for my breakfast smoothie and the last pack of his cigarettes fell out. Those cigarettes have been in there for months and I open the freezer just about every day, but they haven't fallen out before. I thanked John.

A little bit ago, I gathered some things on a tray making a little altar: one of his bandanas, a small urn of his ashes, a picture of the two of us, the small red truck, the pack of cigarettes, and the candle Suwaylu lit when she blessed and anointed his body the day he died. I lit the candle, and took the tray outside, talking to John. I sat for a while, talking to him, then stood and took 10 steps away from the altar. I realized that, in many ways, I have continued walking, because I must, because he's no longer physically here. I turned around and walked back to the altar, sitting and talking some more. I ended with both hands over my heart, telling him I loved him and I always will. And the candle went out. There wasn't any wind or breeze. I took that to mean he heard and accepted my heart's commitment and love.

The weeks leading up to today have been hard, with much grief, which is welcome these days. Like the other firsts so far, the days leading up to the dates were harder than the days themselves.

On Wednesday, the 20th, it will be 8 months since John died: the same amount of time from when the gastroenterologist told John that it looked like he had cancer, until the day John died. Thursday, the 21st, will be our 9th wedding anniversary.

I continue to breathe, to live, to take care of myself, social distancing, isolating myself in our home.

Be well, be safe, dear ones.

Friday, May 22, 2020

Yesterday, our 9th wedding anniversary, I finished putting in my garden and headed back to the house to do something, not paying attention. I walked down a slight incline and the next thing I know, I'm falling, my right foot facing my left leg with an unsettling crack. It hurt! I just wasn't paying attention. Not a new thing these days. Grief brain.

This morning, I knew I needed to get an x-ray. Turns out I fractured the 5th metatarsal in my foot. My back and hips are fine.

Because of the difference in height between the special shoe I need to wear for at least 4 weeks and any of my other shoes, my thigh and butt muscles already hurt so much that walking even a few feet is excruciating. Tylenol helps a bit.

Thursday, June 4, 2020

I saw this rainbow against the dark sky as I was doing my daily walk, grateful my thigh and butt muscles didn't hurt. I talk to John a lot on my walks and this rainbow felt like a confirmation of our continuing connection, even though the world often seems dark to me. Thank you, dear one. I love you.

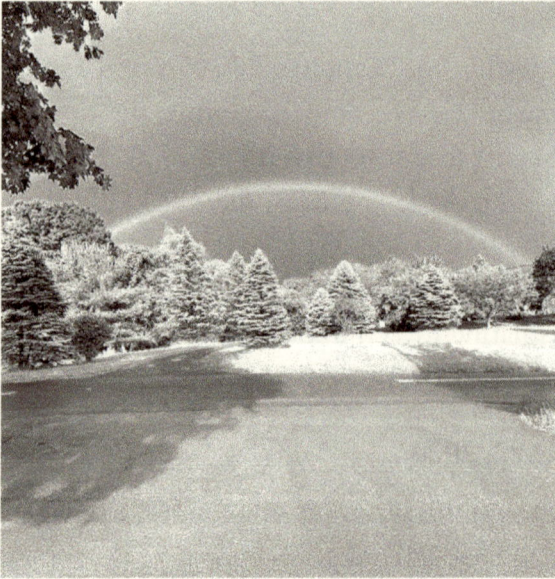

*Rainbow across the road
from the house, 2020*

This rainbow feels like a confirmation from John that he's still around. We both loved the rainbows up here, sharing them every time we saw one.

Tuesday, June 9, 2020

Over the past week or so, I've realized that I feel content, peaceful. Yes, I still miss John. I always will. But it has softened.

Speaking with Margi yesterday, I clarified it. I have had an incredibly blessed life. I've had some challenges, some of them difficult. John's death was the hardest, most painful of them all. Six months after his death, Covid began shutting everything down. I've had some serious conversations with John about his timing, as in "thanks a lot, dude, for skipping out on this one and leaving me here to deal with this by myself."

Then George Floyd was murdered on May 25th. As much as I'd like to be out there, in the protests, I have a fractured foot and I'm in a high risk group for Covid. I've protested before. None of the protests I participated in ever turned violent. Another way I've been blessed in this life. Yet I need to do something!

This takes me right back to something I became aware of some time back: my biggest contribution these days is to be the calm in the storm, the place people can come to talk, the grandmother/elder who invites you to come sit for a cup of tea and then listens, agenda-less.

Another thought came to me as well yesterday: just because a literary agent recommended I write this memoir as auto-fic doesn't mean I have to.

Today, James Kessler's book, *Finding Meaning: The Sixth Stage of Grief* arrived. As I read the first chapter, I knew I needed to sit and begin working with all of the posts and journal entries I've written these past few years as I was John's caregiver, advocate, and mourner. It's felt too hard, too painful. Now it feels right, inside, to embrace and work with whatever this part of my grief process is. I'll discover it later.

There is a small group of us who meet (video only, no audio) every day at 11 Eastern time to write. I haven't been very good at this, like, only once since I was invited three or four weeks ago. Now it feels like the supportive, protective bowl I need to begin this next stage of my grieving.

Early on, I felt I needed to get these posts published as a way to help other caretakers as they live this very difficult and honorable path. I wanted to honor John and his process. Now I'm realizing it's also about honoring *my* path. That whole being blind to the obvious thing. The fact that this on-line writing group exists is yet another way in which I find myself so blessed in this life. Everyone in this group is a writer, most of them published.

And so I pick up the stories, the memories, circling back to the beginning.

Sunday, June 21, 2020

Yesterday marked nine months since John died.

Three quarters of a year. It's still a mix of incredulity and acceptance for me. I've realized there are not only phases of grief, but levels and layers within those phases. The proverbial onion. I'm not sure why this should surprise me, but it does.

My right foot is healing well now, so I don't have to wear the goofy special shoe any more.

It was the first time since John's death when I've needed help getting somewhere. I missed him in a visceral way, in part because I'm not very good at asking for help. And I asked for help.

Earlier last week, I had to have two teeth pulled, one on either side of my upper jaw, both painful and beyond rescue. Because of Covid-19, I'm not sure when it makes sense to get implants, when it will be absolutely safe. I wish John was here so we could talk this through. And laugh. He made me laugh. I get way too serious, all on my own.

Compared to other health issues I've had, these things are pffftttttt minor. One of the inner changes wrought by John's dying and death? My hypochondria is absent. I'm grateful. Life is simpler without it.

Nine months, three of them in relative isolation. The isolation has been an unanticipated blessing. It's given me time to just be by myself, undistracted by busy-ness. I don't have to feel guilty about being alone and actually wanting and appreciating it. That said, Anne driving me to Hagerstown to the orthopedist (and Panera take-out!) was almost like pre-Covid times. Small appreciated gifts in this time.

It's been an eternity and no time at all. I try to remember the days and weeks after he died and they're dim, wrapped up in gauze. I do remember that at the time I thought I was just fine and handling everything very well. I was, for the time.

The phases of grief are a constant learning.

I was on my way to the Farmer's Market this morning. I was driving John's car and sensing all the times he drove it, with his left wrist on the top of the steering wheel, his hand hanging down. My chest felt tight. Checking in, it was love. Huge, huge love for this man who no longer inhabits a physical body. I'm coming to grips with the fact he's never physically going to be here ever again. There are stages to this too, at least for me.

I went back to the orthopedist last Friday. My x-rays show bone growing nicely in the fracture. Since it's not painful, and hasn't been for weeks, I don't need to go back. The big news? I got a script for physical therapy, which they'd said couldn't happen before eight weeks. My back and my muscles are so out of kilter.

Monday, July 20, 2020

Today is ten months since John's death. Like many times these past months, I find myself regretting I scrubbed off the top of the Amazing Grass Superfood canister. John had black Sharpied "Soylent Green" onto the green plastic lid, when we were first exploring pureed foods his stomach would accept. I just couldn't go with the whole soylent green thing. Now? I wish I'd left those Sharpied words there. John wrote them. It was his writing, his sense of humor.

I have kept the two pieces of paper we'd put above the dishwasher to let us know the dishes were clean. One is John's writing, one mine. Except I'm not sure which is which any more. I shake my head at that. How could I not know the difference? It's just one word: "clean" and there are only so many ways a letter can be printed. Or maybe our printing had become similar as we spent more years together. OK?. I'll take that one, true or not. It's comforting.

Thursday, June 25, 2020

Towards the end of the Hospice Grief Group, before Covid, one of the counselors mentioned there were some volunteers who sewed Memory Bears. I decided I'd like four of them. I chose three of John's t-shirts and one of his flannel shirts and took them to Hospice for them to give to the women who make the bears. I asked them to return any leftover material after the bears were made. This was back in maybe January?

Yesterday, I picked up the four memory bears Although I didn't let them know, I was dismayed. They were so stuffed that they were hard. They weren't cuddle-able, at all. I'd thought they could be cuddled. I was nearly in tears. It felt like a sort of betrayal. In truth, it was about my own expectations and not getting more information.

Today, I packaged up and mailed the bears I'd had made for each one of John's three kids. Then, I went through the material they hadn't used when they made the bears. It felt more personal, more John, than I've felt anything in a long while. To see and touch his cut up shirts felt… I don't even have the words right now. I'm in tears, my throat and chest are tight, the world feels heavy and dark. It doesn't help that the news about the pandemic is getting worse, that cases are surging. Knowing that I'll be living like this, essentially alone, for at least a year… today it all feels like too much.

Sunday, August 2, 2020

So many things today.

I did some self-care today. I made dill pickles and pickled beets. The colors are glorious and the flavors will be after they've matured for a few weeks.

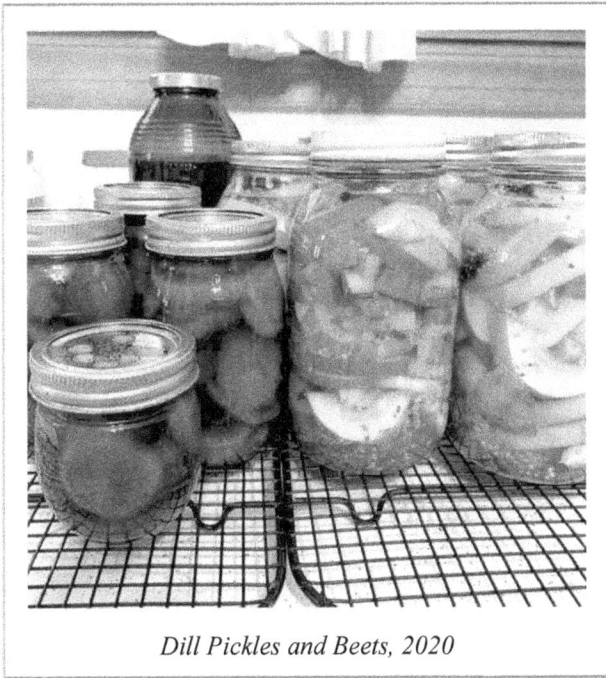

Dill Pickles and Beets, 2020

Cathi, an accomplished musician, recorded *Unchained Melody* by The Righteous Brothers. It was a favorite of mine and of John's. She shared it on my FB page. The comments are healing.

Elmdea: Thank you, Cathi. I miss him more than I have words for and my heart is full 🖤
Cathi: I'm honored to have lifted your spirit today.
Sarah: Cathi… that is so beautiful. It's a haunting version… .
    Cathi: Hmmmm… .good word choice. But that will have to be a private talk sometime.
      Sarah: Cathi yup, yup… .definitely memories abound in your version.
DH: Pletch was our ringleader, more times than I can count. Love the fact that you have protected that memory, regardless of how strangely we have all evolved past those moments. My thanks.
    Elmdea: —and he never stopped being a ringleader… or master storyteller. Your comment brought good memories and a smile. Thank you.
    Cathi: DH, How kind of you to share these thoughts. We shared a deep love while we were romantically together for 8+ important developmental years. Stayed friends till the very end. I will always protect his legacy. I hope you enjoy the song I once recorded for him, and now for Elmdea.

Although we only had 9 years together, John and I had a rare and magical relationship. What I know now is that I'm still here because there's something else I'm to do with my life, part of which is honoring John's legacy of love and wisdom. I hope you're able to find that, too. It's hard. And it's love.

Wednesday, August 5, 2020

I've joined a 30 day writing prompts group around grief. I've no idea where this will take me or if it's even the right time for this. Whatever. I'm giving it a go. Here's my first bit of writing.

The person I used to be had finally found her perfect companion and mate. She knew this and was grateful, rarely taking it for granted. She and John had waited until their early

60's to finally find each other. It was magical and scary… and it worked.

We felt like we'd been comfortably married for decades, and we never even reached one decade together. We loved each other as is, the perfect parts and the parts that drove us nuts. We had each other's backs. We were looking forward to growing older together, secure and safe in our love. We talked about all kinds of things, bouncing ideas off each other, trying to make sense of the world around us, all the while knowing we were good where we were. Pre John's dying and death, I was quite focused on my own health, because of my health issues, which are now, thankfully, resolved. I was excited and diligent about doing my physical therapy and exploring new ways to be active in the world. My back surgery was healing, tho not as quickly as I wanted. After? Pffffttt.

One of the biggest differences now from then is the lack of fear I have when the house makes noises, inside or out. I was hypervigilant for years because of break-ins thirty plus years ago. Now? Whatever. For a while, all I could remember was the horror of watching him being eaten alive by the cancer. Now I'm starting to remember the times before: the laughter, the deep discussions, the teasing, the brilliance of his quirky mind. And it's memory. It isn't current reality. It isn't who I am now. I'm unsure who I am now.

The only thing I know for sure is I've been broken open. It was his last gift to me, one I would gladly have done without… and one I choose to accept and honor.

Thursday, August 6, 2020

In this morning's email was one from Penzey's Spices. They are giving away some Hug Blankets and asking people to nominate someone (or themselves) for one. They are colorful and they really look like a hug. So, I've nominated myself.

When they asked me why I could use a hug, I wrote this:

"My beloved husband died September 20, 2019. It was just us. I'm in my upper 60's with no family close and hugs are nearly non-existent so touch hunger is a very real thing for me."

Friday, August 7, 2020

Before John's cancer and death, I thought grief was something you worked through, learned and grew from, and it went away. I figured if I honored and expressed my anticipatory grief when it welled up, side-swiped me, leveled me, then my grief after his death would be easier to handle, swifter to heal. Hah! What I know now, nearing eleven months after his death, is that grief shifts and changes, it has phases, new depths and new heights, and it's unmistakably my grief for John.

My grief isn't as raw, as sharp as it was those months when he was actively dying and after his death. There's relief that it *isn't* going away. It's settled in, much the way a new shoe forms to your foot through daily use. I've discovered a dearness, a sweetness to my evolving grief. "Dear" and "sweet" aren't words I've ever associated with grief. Yet that's how it feels, at least lately.

There are days when grief whomps me upside the head. There are days when grief's more in the background. Always, it's present. I don't need to search for it. It's part of who I am, of who I'm becoming, whoever that person is/will be. Always, now, grief is welcome. It isn't going to disappear on me. I'm grateful.

My grief has been a mostly solitary journey, partly by choice, partly imposed. I'm probably one of the few who's actually grateful for the self-isolation that Covid has required. It's meant (and continues to mean) that I don't have to justify my need for solitude to folk who don't understand.

Not every loss is the same. When my father died, I had one deep sob and a few days of tears. We weren't close, he was an alcoholic, and he was a misogynist. I think that brief grief was more for the father I didn't have than the one I did.

Talking to my mom and my sister, neither of them have experienced this kind of grief. They've no idea what I'm attempting to convey to them. I've let it go. There's no point. They have no direct experience, so no direct understanding. It's not right or wrong. It's just how life works.

I had months of grieving before John died. I hid that anticipatory grief as much as possible from him. He could "read" me well before the cancer, chemo, pain, and constant nausea required his focus. We would have brief conversations, but his attention was fleeting. In many ways, it felt like he'd already died.

Saturday, August 8, 2020

Where I live is both familiar and unknown. No, it isn't a paradox. The house, its furnishings, our cars, these are unchanged.

I live in the same 1940's house John and I lived in. I pass the living room where the hospital bed was, where he died, every day. Whenever I think of moving, the place I dream of looks a lot like this one, so I'll stay a while longer. I'm sometimes surprised when a background object is suddenly visible, like his wooden back-scratcher hanging along the door frame.

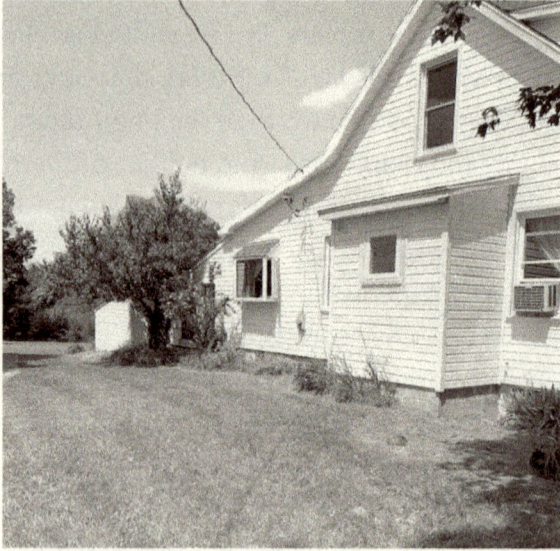

Our 1940s house, 2020

The house is quieter now. The low sounds of battle in the MMO's he played, 1960's ballads he loved, his voice, are dim echoes in memory. And the silence of no conversation. We had so many, about so many things.

On my walks on the country road beside our house, I watch leaves turning in the wind, dragon's-breath fogs rising from the hollows after sunrise, the clouds. I talk to John a lot on these walks. I know he can't see any of this. He'll never see any of it again, not in my lifetime. Or maybe he can see it a little through my eyes. I like to imagine that now and again. These walks are when I feel closest to him, when there's only sky above, like that somehow makes it easier to reach him. It brings home, yet again, how he's not here to see the things I see; that life really does continue after death. It isn't dependent on our seeing of it.

Most of all, I don't understand why I'm still here, why I'm watching and breathing the changing of seasons, why I'm still alive. There must be a reason for it. At least I want there to be a reason. I miss him so much.

Sunday, August 9, 2020

You didn't wear any cologne. Dr. Bronner's Peppermint Castile Soap, that you used when you showered, doesn't leave much of a scent. The only thing I have that really carries your smell, faintly, is the pillow you rested your legs on, those last months of your life, when cancer, the chemo, and the radiation were wreaking havoc on your body.

There is one other thing: incense. You'd burn half a stick or so each morning as you did your morning prayers and meditated. You had some favorites: Astha, Sun, Midnight. The Dragon's Blood was for festivals, camping with friends.

Super Hit. That was the one I burned in the living room, the last 10 days of your life, when you were bed-bound after your fall, no longer able to get to the smoking porch. You still wanted your cigarettes, but not as often. Winston's, in the red box. I didn't want the living room smelling like cigarette smoke. I didn't think I could handle that after you died. I knew you were dying, and I was still in some denial.

The caretakers would burn the incense, too, then put it out when you'd finished smoking. I was grateful to them. I didn't know caretakers would take care of me, too, like making sure I was eating. I didn't know I needed that. I knew I couldn't lift you or shift you. I was still healing from back surgery a year and a half earlier. I couldn't remember to do my physical therapy, to strengthen my core. Everything was focused on you.

This morning, I decided to burn some of that incense. Just smelling the Super Hit in its box, unlit, brought back those days. And your last morning. The power of memory and scent.

Looking Back

The first year after John's death took me six months into the pandemic. I had planned to get together with a number of people and this couldn't happen. I wanted to visit with John Sr. and Ero. I wanted to meet Cathi. I wanted to see Mara. I wanted time with my friends. None of that could happen during lockdown. Some of it never did.

I read and I read and I read. There were a few novels, but most were spiritual books, primarily about life after death. Some were written in the late 1800's, some in the last few years. I needed confirmation that what I know, deep inside, is true. There is life after death and John is alive and well, in a different form, on the "other side." Some of those books are listed in the back under Resources.

Being unable to get together with people who had known John caused such great pain. I could not share stories and memories, we couldn't hug each other. This is necessary for closure and the pandemic denied me this.

I have no idea how the millions of people who lost loved ones during the pandemic coped with the isolation, the lack of funeral or memorial gatherings, and the utter horror of that time. Yes, we all managed, but at a price that only we know.

We made it through, most of us. I'm grateful for that. I'm grateful John died before Covid hit because I can't imagine how much more difficult his care would have been, how much more isolated we both would have been. My heart cries for those of you who had to navigate the dying and deaths of your loved ones during the pandemic years.

PART X:
COMING UP ON THE FIRST ANNIVERSARY

Monday, August 10, 2020

Over this past day, I've sat with Grief, wondering what I would write. She (figuratively) tapped me on my shoulder. *"Share the collage."* she said. *"That's when you began your process of accepting me, instead of hoping I'd go away."*

Ah.

She's been my companion since February 15, 2019, the day we got John's Stage IV Esophageal cancer diagnosis.

Over the course of my life, I've learned that the only way forward with hard inner work and emotion is to welcome it whenever it shows up. If I don't, I would feel WAY worse when it finally broke through.

I wasn't up for worse. Nope, no way, Nopity-nope-nope.

There were times when I couldn't, because, whether it was the right thing or not, I tried to protect John from as much of my grief as I could. I know I didn't fool him, but he had his own work he was doing: meeting his own death and saying goodbyes to his kids and his 97 year old father.

I created the collage / watercolor December 16, 2019, 4 days shy of the 3 month anniversary of John's death.

She and I are good friends at this point, maybe even best friends. We're growing and learning together. She has distinct phases, rising out of the one before. She's gentler now, in her own fierce way. I welcome her, without apology or resistance. She's an intrinsic part of my life and will be until I take my last breath. I'm grateful for her presence and her (sometimes tough) love.

The upper left is how I was feeling when I created this

collage. Lots of questions, lots of tears, tearing pain. The lower right was where I hoped I could be/grow to at some point.

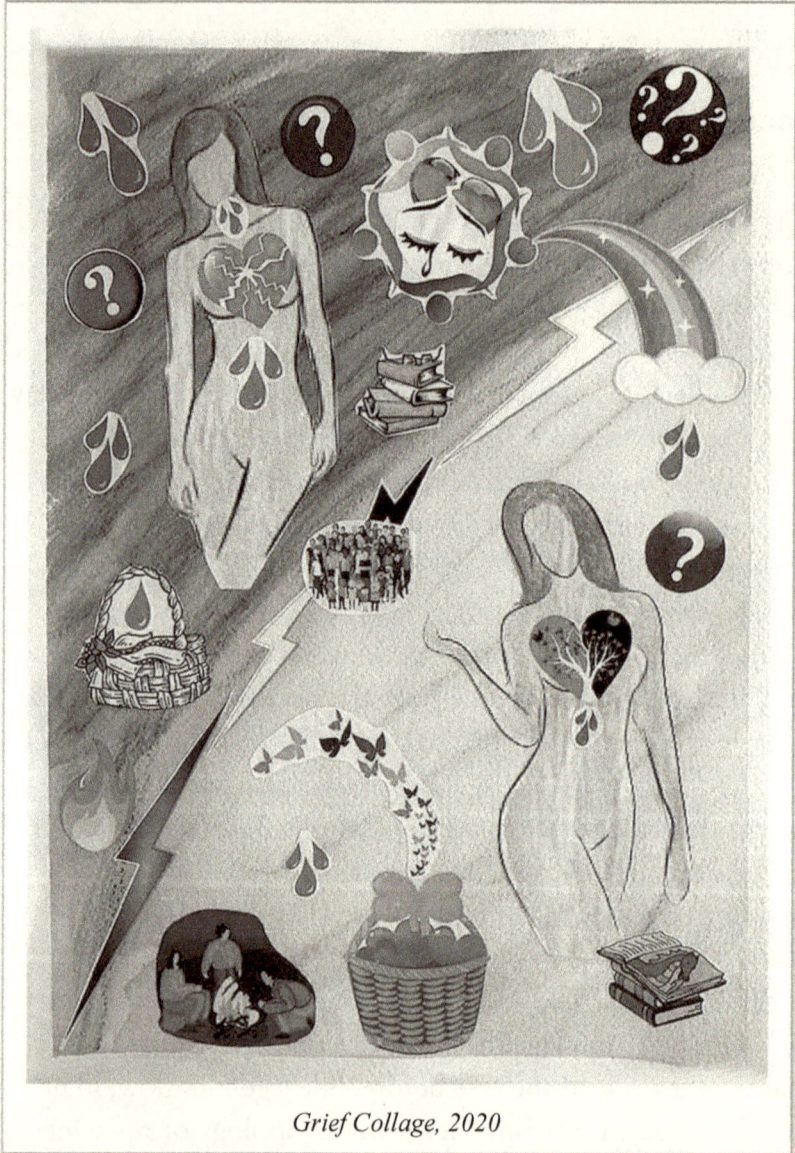

Grief Collage, 2020

What I knew then and I know now is the only thing that can help me get through the lightning bolts is a community of people, and hope (the rainbow). I'm making some progress. The lower right portion is still a dream, but I've had hints. As I sit here typing this, it dawns on me that she and I will create another collage: of our evolving relationship, of transitional spaces.

I'm leaving out more description, because I want to leave space for what does (or doesn't) speak to you, my fellow grief writing group members. It's another thing I've learned over the course of my life (and Grief is reinforcing this): leave room for other explanations and meanings.

Thursday, August 13, 2020

I've spent a few days on this prompt, mulling it over. This one felt like it needed /requested I spend more time with it. So I have.

Turns out part of my kindness is allowing myself to "fall behind", not staying current with the daily prompts, catching up as I can.

The recurrent theme these past days has been allowing myself to look at my habits, patterns, and ways of doing things at home. How many were made to accommodate John, both before his illness and then when I became his caretaker? None of them were what I would call major life changes. They were part of the little compromises that we both made as we created and evolved our lives together.

One is where I meditate. John was an early riser and I'm not. So I began meditating in bed, rather than downstairs. It was quieter. I wasn't distracted by him getting coffee or whatever. He didn't have to worry about disturbing me. It was a win-win. Now? It doesn't matter and I still meditate in bed. Now I'm giving it some thought. As a result, as a kindness to myself, rather than preserving a habit created when John and I lived together, I'll begin experimenting with where else (and when else) I'll meditate each day.

Why, I ask, is this a kindness to myself? Hmmmm. I'm still figuring out who I am in the world without John physically here. I get hints of his spirit / soul now and again, but he's not physically here. My kindness to myself is permission to explore doing things differently and then go with what feels best for now, knowing it may well change again, rather than holding on to what became jointly created patterns. Some will remain, some will shift, some will fade.

My kindness to myself is to accept, yet again (and again, and again) that things change. Holding on to what was doesn't serve.

Friday, August 14, 2020

There are two people now who are guiding stars to me as I travel this path of grieving. One is my Hospice grief counselor (who I continue to see). Again and again, she has assured me that I'm normal, I'm not crazy. That grief is like this. That there really isn't a set way to grieve. We all share the anguish, the wordlessness of it. We experience and express it in our individual ways.

The other is the Hospice Chaplain who came to see John many times in his last weeks. Chaplain W. lost his wife 9 years ago. He's now doing Hospice work. He's very good. Our conversation at the wake, where he said that widow is an honorable title, has stuck with me. I'm slowly making peace with being "a widow."

I have some fictional guides. Currently, they are the heroines in Tamora Pierce's books. They rise, in a very patriarchal world. They rise. Another is Menolly, in the *Dragonsong* books by Anne McCaffrey. She, too, rises.

I, too, shall rise, grief as my companion, befriended. Moment by moment. Step by step.

Saturday, August 15, 2020

I highlighted words and phrases that jumped off the page at me from a travel magazine.

You loved the water. It refreshed you. You dreamt of a house on the beach, where you could stay in the comfort of your place.

Coming up on the first anniversary of your death, I'm in a redesign of my life, unwanted though that is. I'm seeking something iconic, with a measure of safety, which I can't take lightly. A natural area with a powerful waterfall, a lovely waterfront, and the cool waters of a lake certainly meets the iconic part. It would be lovely to travel with friends to this unknown place. Perhaps it's in my imagination.

Sunday, August 16, 2020

Today's grief prompt was to write about a grief within my grief.

Your red plaid shirt was your favorite. You wore it so often, you blew out an elbow and it was faded from so many washings. You still insisted on wearing it. It was broken in, perfect. Now… now you're no longer here to wear it. I touch its softness. Your scent is long gone because it was washed for the last time in late winter, after we'd gotten your diagnosis. I still had no real idea how important things like that would be to me, after your death.

Hospice has a volunteer who makes memory bears. Oh yes! To have a bear made from that shirt that I could hold. I got it back many months later. It was awful. It wasn't cuddly or cute. It had button eyes attached to each other through the head so they pulled its face inward, and buttons on arms and legs so they could move. Great for a toy, but not for cuddling. It still hurts, what was done to your shirt. I can't bear to throw it away either.

Your favorite red flannel shirt. Maybe there's enough of it left for a real memory bear, a cuddle-able one.

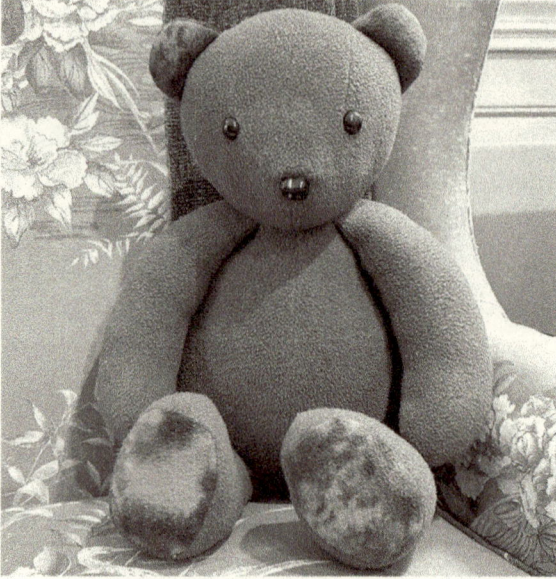

A Cuddly Memory Bear made later from John's favorite Polar Fleece

Monday, August 17, 2020

As far back as I can remember, I've been aware of inequities and the destructiveness of the human animal on the environment. I've also been incredibly naive. To handle the pain of the inequities, I learned early on to compartmentalize them. Now I'm working with my therapist to open up those compartments, giving them air and light. It's part of honoring my grief for John breaking me open. It's a process, not an overnight sort of thing.

Wednesday, August 19, 2020

I was John's sole caregiver until the last 10 days of his life. There were days when I got REALLY angry, yelling / screaming angry. So angry I had to go to the garage to scream, so he wouldn't hear. I felt guilty I was angry at him / the situation. I wanted my life back. And I knew, at a deep, pre-verbal level, it wasn't coming back.

The hospice social worker told me my anger was reasonable and I'd handled it well. She would know. She went on to say that the key was that I wasn't acting on it. Other than screaming in the garage, I wasn't.

Thing is, me and anger have never been buddies. I'm not good with it, my own or others.

Losing John... the hardest part was watching him diminish before my eyes. It hurt more than anything I'd felt before. To witness cancer eating him alive, literally. That was anguish beyond words. I'd try to imagine how it felt for him and I couldn't. Yes, I'd had my own brush with death four years earlier (pericarditis) and made peace with it. But to live with constant nausea and pain and know it was never going away, that only death would bring release?

And yet how many times a day did I pause on my way past the living room, waiting, to make sure he took his next breath? Multiple times for months. I was never ready for him to go, not even when he did.

The anger is past. Now there is grief, a strange peace, the disconnection from each day, the surreal aspect of still being alive, that Covid has amplified.

Thursday, August 20, 2020

Today, August 20, marks eleven months since your death. It seems like forever and no time at all. I'm still here in our house. I know I told you I wasn't sure how long I'd stay. Now I know.

I'm staying here for a bit, probably years. And not just because of the pandemic (which I'm grateful you missed, but damn I wish you were here, healthy).

Although we only had 9 years together, you and I had a rare and magical relationship. I keep coming back to knowing that I'm still here because there's something else I'm to do with my life. I still don't know what.

You never really got to see the house after the siding was completed. The one time I got you outside to see the progress, you quietly asked me what you were looking at. I told you. You said "Oh. It looks nice." It was two months before your death.

Every time I look at the house now, I think of you. Of how hard you worked to make sure everything would be settled and in place for me. You were already exhausted by the esophageal cancer and your inability to eat. Thank you with all of my heart and more. My years with you were the best years of my life. That's a big part of why I want to stay here. I want to be able to touch the memories, stop in certain spots and remember a hug, a laugh...

There have been some changes. I now have an LP fueled generator hooked up to a special fuse box in case the electricity goes out. I don't have to worry about pull-starting the old generator and stringing all those reeeaalllyyyy long extension cords through the house. It's a relief. Solar was just not in the cards, much as I would have liked it.

Another change is the dining room table. You would laugh. Boy would you laugh! Yeah, I used to bug you to clear off the accumulated piles of mail, books, and who knows what else behind the lazy susan. You called yourself my chaos coach. You still are. Me, who had to have the dining room table cleared off every few weeks? Wellllll... the main clear spot these days is where I sit to eat. The rest is things like books, papers I need to put somewhere else, and stuff on its way from one place to another, which sometimes takes days. Since it's just me, it doesn't matter how soon it moves along.

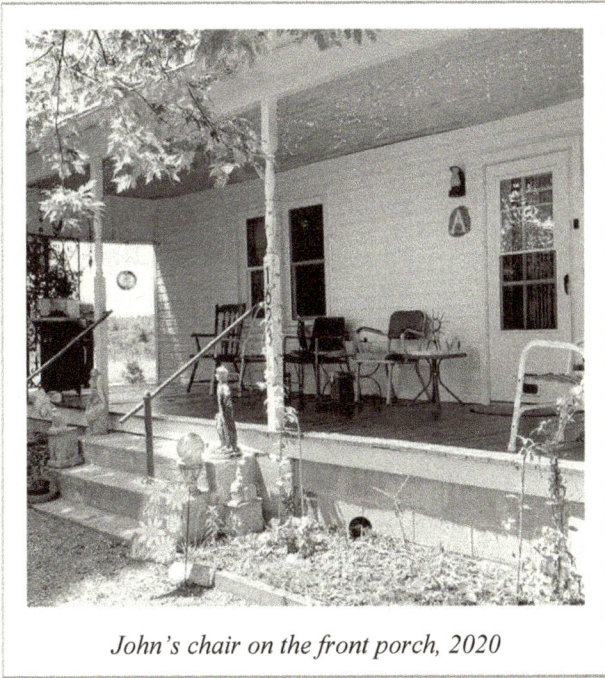

John's chair on the front porch, 2020

I miss you. I wish you were here, sitting on the front porch in your tan chair, waving at the folks driving by, watching the sunrise, drinking your coffee. I wish you were here to enjoy the improvements you got started before you died. I wish you were here.

Friday, August 21, 2020

I breathe into my grief, which has felt absent for several days. And there it is. Tears rise, my chest tightens, and there's a knot in my throat. I'm relieved. I was beginning to wonder if I didn't even belong in this group of grief writers, if I'd somehow lost my grief or I'd pushed it away too well.

Such a difference from early on, when grief was ALL there was. Now, it has softened to a welcome ache, its own presence. At least today.

I'm coming up on some big one year anniversaries in September: the day he asked Hospice for a hospital bed, the day he fell (and was bed-bound after that), and… the morning he took his last breath, as I held his hand and cupped his cheek. Many days of this next month will be hard, probably harder than the actual anniversary days. At least that's how it's been for the other one year anniversaries so far.

I'm grateful grief is still here, that it continues its ever evolving process of holding me, sometimes demanding my attention, sometimes giving me space to breathe. I'm grateful for the comfort of its now familiar presence: the ache, the tightness, the tears, the being-ness.

I'm grateful for the small things I can touch to check-in with grief: his watch that's still running, the last wad of bills he took out of his pocket, the empty box of his last pack of cigarettes and one crushed cigarette butt, his back scratcher hanging on the door frame…

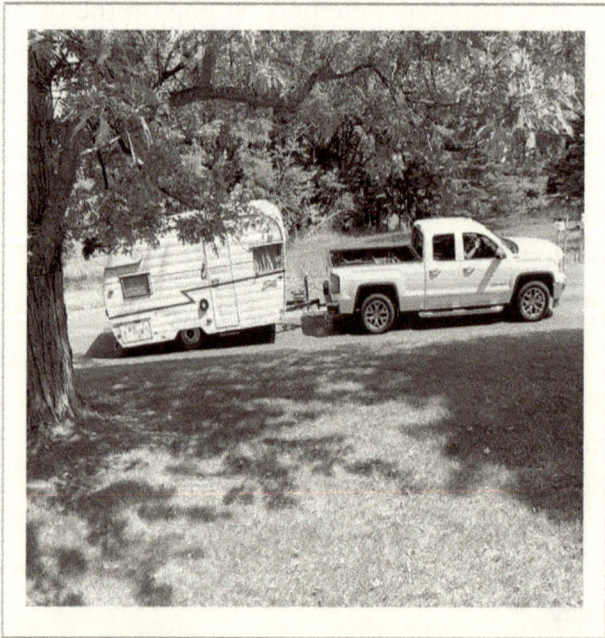

And today, John, I sold your 1963 Shasta Airflyte trailer. You were so tickled to have it. You would pull it up to where you wanted to be, put up the awning, take out the chairs, string some blue twinkle lights and you were done. We had thought about restoring it but I just can't. Without you here, I'm not interested. The woman who bought it will be restoring it, so I'm glad we kept it safe for her.

Saturday, August 22, 2020

My grief and my knowledge of grief are often an unwanted guest. I'm amazed at how differently each of us can mourn, depending on who we are and our relationship with the one who died. My grief is welcome in some small circles where tenderness is alive.

An empath, I've learned when and how to shield myself. That skill has been very helpful as I mourn my beloved. I'm seen as being helpful, non-judgmental, and supportive. When I'm the one needing that, there are few who can or will meet me. It's no one's fault. It's just how it works out. This kind of grief can't really be imagined, it can only be experienced.

Saturday, August 23, 2020

This opportunity to explore my grief through the prompts has been more of a gift than I'd anticipated. Much of the writing happens in my head before I even sit down to type it. And I've been discovering resistance, which I didn't anticipate.

Or maybe it isn't resistance so much as it's a need to let the feelings and thoughts sit, meander, coalesce, find their voice. My grief has entered yet another phase, a phase that is softer, where I feel John's presence more as a comfort and his absence less, because he's here, just differently. Our hearts are well and truly connected. We have each other's backs physically and non-physically. It just manifests differently than it did. Writing has helped that clarify and grow.

Monday, August 24, 2020

Before writing this, I sat and centered myself, eyes closed, feeling my heart (both literal and figurative), my fingers on my keyboard. I've cleaned up some misspellings, and this is what I saw / came to me. It wasn't what I anticipated.

Unexpectedly, a black hole emerges to my inner eye. OK. I can be with this. As I sit, I begin to see small pinpricks of light. I'm drawn closer to this dark, unknown vastness that is my heart and the pinpricks become larger, become stars. I'm surrounded by them. I'm not alone. I'm part of them.

OK.

Breathe.

That's the truth of my Spirit heart. What about my human heart?

It's a little wobbly, unsteady, wistful, feeling compressed into my chest. I sold the 1963 Shasta trailer yesterday. It was a project we were going to work on, then cancer came calling. A dream, gone, waved down the road. Gone with someone who will bring that dream into her reality.

Both the space of all the stars and the wistful heart are together, both at the same time. Both are real. Both are valid.

Breathe.

The darkness and the stars begin to wrap themselves around my hurting human heart. Shall I let it? Do I have a choice? Yes, I do.

The heart of my spirit enfolds my human heart of grief and holds it in love. It's allowing deeper breaths. There is a mild peace alongside the grief and the everydayness of doing things that still being alive require. It's a welcome easing, without erasure.

Thank you.

Thursday, August 27, 2020

Bit of a rant here. There are memes that show up talking about how happiness is something we can create and grief passes, it isn't a permanent resident. I'm finding this true about the happiness, some days.

And at the same time, who the hell's life is that anyway? Platitudes I'm uninterested in hearing.

And saying grief isn't a permanent resident in my life dismisses me, my feelings, my life, now and going forward. I am the primary residence for my grief, just as I am the primary residence for my love for John. My grief and my love are roommates, life-long at this point, interdependent.

My experience of life has been expanded to include this deep grief and its evolution as the days and months pass. There are moments when I don't feel grief. That or I've become so used to its residence that it's just part of my day, until it taps (or punches) me, reminding me, yet again, that it is indeed a permanent resident.

And make no mistake, it *is* reassuring when my grief demands my attention. Early on, not so much because it was all there was and it was hard to breathe, think, not dissociate. Then, I wanted it "healed and gone."

Now I know it never will be. It's now intrinsic to who I am. I'm beyond good with that. I'm grateful, odd as that may sound.

Monday, August 31, 2020

Today, I went to Hagerstown for my endoscopy / colonoscopy. Anne offered to drive me. In the past, I didn't have to arrange that sort of thing. John and I drove each other where we needed to go.

The hardest thing about today? Not the prep, unpleasant as that always is. It was when I was going over the paperwork and there was the question of who to notify in case of any emergency.

Oooof. It took my breath away.

Almost a year later and… it hits me once again. John isn't here. He can't be notified. I ended up putting the name of my friend, who also has my Medical Power of Attorney. It hadn't even occurred to me I'd need to be changing that.

Monday, September 7, 2020

Self care has come up multiple times this week. I had to ask my grief counselor to help me identify things that would be self care. And then I asked my therapist.

Why now? Today, September 7, is 13 days until the first anniversary of your death. This past week or so, I've found myself in tears. Coming on your wallet unexpectedly. Going for an endoscopy/colonoscopy that was postponed while you were sick and then dying. A friend fixing me cinnamon rolls and realizing I felt nurtured, which I haven't felt for too long. Buying a new gas stove because the old one is getting dangerous. And knowing how you made do again and again and again in your life, like you weren't deserving of more.

Realizing that I've given very little thought to my life beyond this first year. I'm past trying to anticipate what will bring tears. These past few weeks, they've been nearly as frequent as they were in the first weeks and months after your death, minus the searing, sharp, take-my-breath-away pain.

For these next weeks, I'll do my best to take at least one walk a day, often talking to you. I'll sit on the front porch for fifteen minutes and just look, hear, and watch. There's always something since our house is in the country. I may use Thich Nhat Hanh's book *How To Sit* to give me some structure while I sit. I'll skip reading the news. I'm putting aside the non-fiction books and focusing on reading for pleasure.

I'll plan what I want to do on September 21st, when it will be a year and a day. I'm reminding myself there's a reason why "a year and a day" is so often referenced in the old tales and rituals. I'll plan something opposite for the 22nd, so I don't get stuck. Loving myself, I give myself permission to switch things around.

I'm letting go of feeling like I have to hurry and finish all the grief writing prompts. I just can't right now. And that's ok. That's as it is and as my grief needs it to be. All of this is. All of this is. *crying*

This is loving myself in gentle action.

Wednesday, September 9, 2020

Last night, I was awakened by a sound. I realized what I'd heard was a thump and an animal cry, possibly a deer. There was a car stopped and a woman (I could hear her voice, not her words) was apparently looking around on the road. I heard a car door close and they drove on.

This morning, I got up and looked out my back upstairs window. There was a deer lying down in the grass on the lawn. It was alert, head up, ears twitching. It tried to get up. It couldn't. It appeared both front legs were broken. How it got 100+ feet from the road… shock I guess. I called the county and they sent out a Sheriff's Deputy to put it down. One shot. Before they got here, I spent some time sending peace / comfort to the deer. No idea if it helped… either of us.

This is the first time this has happened to me: a mortally injured deer in my yard.

This has shaken me for two reasons: the suffering of the deer and the fact that tonight is the first anniversary of when John fell. After that, he needed help getting out of the bed to smoke or use the urinal. And a few days after that he was bed bound until his death on the 20th.

I'm grateful I have a session with Margi today!

Saturday, September 19, 2020

Tomorrow is the first anniversary of John's death and my grief counselor suggested I plan some things for tomorrow and the next few days.

Tomorrow will be pretty quiet for me. I'll need it.

Monday (year and a day), I'll be doing more around the house, still by myself.

Tuesday, I want to do things with friends, as a way to say I want more interaction and active community in this coming year.

Saturday, September 19, 2020

Cathi: Tomorrow (September 20, 2020) will be John's first Yarzheit… Yiddish word for the anniversary of his death. My heart is filled with love and grace and gratitude for a life interestingly led… and the friendship it has brought us this year.

Elmdea: I, too, am grateful for the friendship John brought us. It doesn't seem real that tomorrow is the 20th and he'll have been gone a year.

Sunday, September 20, 2020

The house is filled with the smell of a pot roast, slowly cooking in the crock-pot. It's been about two years since I last fixed one. It was one of John's favorite meals. I thawed out, heated, and ate the leftovers of that last pot roast months after John died, crying as I did. I don't believe there will be tears today… and I'll find out.

It's been a blessed day. The days and weeks leading up to today were hard, almost as hard as just after John died.

Today I woke up early, lit a candle, and spent some time with the memorial poster I made for his wake and his service. Then I sat outside, watching the sunrise and talking to him. At the end, a three point buck walked across the yard and then across the road. I haven't seen him before. I took it as a message from John that he's with me.

Later, Cathi and I spoke and I learned the story of the toy red truck. I'm keeping those details in my heart. The story itself was a further gift from John, a year after he left his body. I feel very loved. One of the many gifts from John has been this friendship between Cathi and me. We were the relationship bookends of John's adult life.

John's love is present in my heart. It feels like enough right now.

Looking Back

Step by step, I made it through the first year of my grief for John.

The down side was the Pandemic, which isolated me. While that isolation made some things easier, it reinforced my already introverted nature. I didn't have to pretend I was ok.

The upside was Zoom, which was so much easier for me than other video platforms. I could "see" my therapist, Margi. I could "go" to physical therapy. I could consult my doctor.

Wearing N95 masks, I could get my broken foot taken care of and get my endoscopy/colonoscopy.

John Sr. and Ero were at the beach house because it was safer for them there than in their DC condo. It was four hours away and I'd become so reclusive that driving any distance felt overwhelming. In retrospect, my reclusion was how I managed the impact of grief in isolation. I'm still learning how to re-engage with the world.

PART XI:
YEAR TWO

Tuesday, September 29, 2020

Well, I can now positively confirm that there is no magical healing of grief after getting through the first year. Grief is still here. I'm feeling sort of let down. I thought the grief would feel just a little lighter. It doesn't.

Culturally, the focus is on the first year and all those first anniversaries. After that? Not much is spoken of. A century or more ago, women wore black for a year after the death of a family member. For the second year, they wore gray and, perhaps, dull lavender. It was a signal that they were grieving. I'm sure it was a mixed blessing for many. Scarlet O'Hara comes to mind.

Monday, October 5, 2020

While I've made a great deal of peace with John's death and his very permanent absence, today I was reminded of the futility of trying to avoid grief triggers. It's also the one year anniversary of his memorial service. I haven't really felt much one way or the other about this particular first.

John had an office chair that he wore out and replaced, but didn't want to get rid of. Then, when he was sick, then dying, he had me bring it to the smoking porch for him to sit it. It worked there. Since his death, it's been sitting in storage because it was so big. He was 6'3" and 277 pounds pre-cancer.

Last week, I had a brilliant idea: call the trash service and see if they would pick up the old falling apart grill and that office chair. I was told "Yes, just leave it out on Monday with your regular trash."

Yesterday afternoon, I dug the chair out. I sat in it for a while, running my hands on the arms where he'd completely worn off the covering. My feet didn't touch the ground and the chair was uncomfortable. No, there was no reason to keep it.

I heard the trash truck around 7 this morning. I got up and looked out the window. The grill was already gone. What I saw was the last bit of the bottom wheels on his chair going in and being compacted.

It's destroyed and gone. Like John. There's no retrieving it or getting it back. Like John. I had no idea seeing that chair go would bring tears and grief back up. I breathe, reminding myself that this may happen many times over the rest of my life.

Sunday, October 25, 2020

A meme showed up today. It captures my experience of the pandemic so far coupled with grief and the losing of days, time, thoughts, memory (otherwise known as grief brain). It makes as much sense.

"If 2020 was a math problem: If you're walking on the ice cream at 5 ounces per toaster and your bicycle loses a sock, how much gravy will you need to repaint your hamster?"

Tuesday, October 27, 2020

A package from Penzey's Spices arrived in the mail today. It didn't make sense because I haven't ordered anything from them in months. But my name was on the address label. On opening it, I found a blanket, the Penzey's Hug Blanket. It's beautiful bright colors with hands embracing the word "HUG".

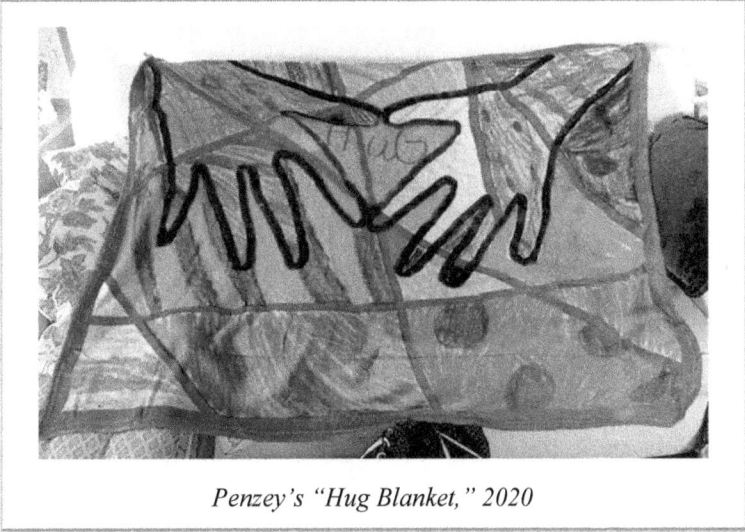

Penzey's "Hug Blanket," 2020

I'd forgotten that in August I'd put my name in for one of the free ones they were giving away to those who need a hug. My reason was that I'd lost John and I'm now alone, isolating during this pandemic. I wrapped it around myself and cried. I'll be sending them a thank you note.

Sunday, November 1, 2020

I've found, for me, that a "thick skin" makes things worse because it keeps my own stuff in that needs out, as well as shutting others out. Even in grief, I've paradoxically found that allowing my own grief and vulnerability out, I'm less vulnerable. A paradox.

I read *The Wild Edge of Sorrow* by Francis Weller shortly after John died and found it helpful, in part because he addresses so many different types of grief. I was particularly struck by grief for our environment / planet because that is part of my grief.

One of (many) aspects that appealed to me was the grief ritual he offers. At the time I read it, I needed a place for my grief to be heard, for my story to be heard. John's death was foremost, and the changes I've personally witnessed and experienced in the climate also needed voice. *The Wild Edge of Sorrow* brought those two together for me so I could begin another level of my grief process. It will be ongoing, the proverbial onion with many layers.

Tuesday, November 3, 2020

There are times when I wonder if I imagined the whole thing because it doesn't feel "real" anymore. Which, in this moment and all the rest of the moments in my life, is true. John is now memories, no longer my current reality. It's mind-boggling.

Thursday, November 5, 2020

I took a new selfie today. It's been maybe two years since I've done that. What I notice is how much I've aged. That's no surprise, it has been a rough few years.

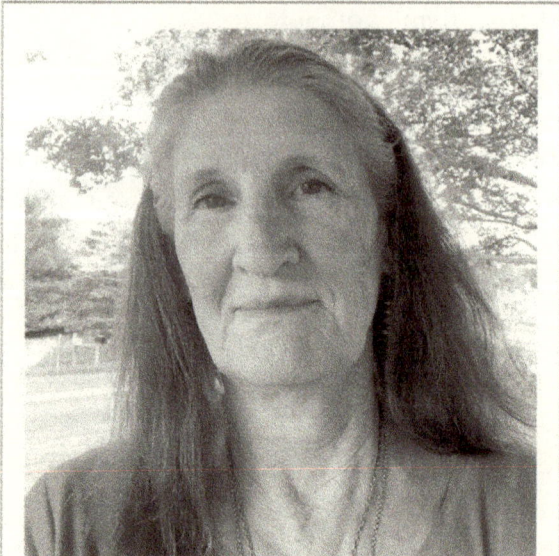

Elmdea, 2020

Friday, November 13, 2020

I'm finding myself nearly in tears a lot today. I'm just missing him so much. Not that I haven't been, but it's been more background than foreground since his first death day anniversary, which was one month and twenty-four days ago.

Lately, I've been regretting cleaning up his room so quickly after he died. At the time, I just had to do it. Now I wonder if it was a way to try and wipe out a lot of the visual cues of his absence, my own form of denial. If his room didn't look like his room anymore, then I could look at it without being triggered. I'm not even sure that makes sense, but then grief doesn't, I've learned and continue to learn. I read about people who, for years, leave a loved one's room just as they left it. I never thought I'd say this, but I really miss his clutter. It drove me nuts when he was alive and now? Now, I miss it.

I have more memories of John's and my time before he became ill. This past year was about the trauma of watching him ravaged by the cancer and his dying. It was like those 11 months usurped all the memories of our time before.

Now... I feel like I'm able to reclaim our prior life, both ordinary and non-ordinary. As such, my grief feels less like it's ripping and tearing and more like a growing tenderness, the way a physical wound can be tender. My grief isn't less, it's different. I'll take this reclaiming of earlier memories over the tearing anguish of the trauma. It's gentle love expressing, rather than fierce love tearing.

Monday, November 23, 2020

So. A number of people in the Writing Your Grief Alumni group have mentioned rage. I shrugged and moved on. It didn't relate to my grief experience. Until today.

Ever since he died, I've wanted to be in contact with John, to have conversations. That came pretty close to happening yesterday, but I felt a heaviness, a resistance inside. It was a bad day anyway. I'm just not caring about much.

This morning? I had a fit of screaming rage. "Why the hell couldn't you get a f'ing endoscopy!?! If you had, you'd probably still be here and I wouldn't be doing this whole pandemic thing all by myself. I asked you to a bunch of times. A bunch. But noooo, you wouldn't listen. And that choice you made? That's left me here, by myself, during a pandemic."

I remember early on, after you'd been diagnosed, realizing that you hadn't been upfront with me about how you were feeling physically. At the time, it helped, because that was your choice and there wasn't anything I could / would feel guilty about.

Today? I'm really pissed. How dare you! Your decision not only killed you, it's left me here alone. You'd asked me, several months before you died, if I had any unresolved issues with you. At the time, I didn't. Today? You bet I do! Oh yes! I'm not sure how this will all work out, but for now, I'm just pissed and I'm staying that way until I'm not.

Monday, February 1, 2021

Its gently snowing here. We'll have maybe 10" by tomorrow morning when it's done. I'm delighting in the beauty of the little icicles, the snow covered branches of the Rose of Sharon, and the purple stained glass Healing bindrune my sister made me.

I'm grateful I can take joy in the small things. And that I've found someone who will plow out my driveway! There's no way I can shovel all of that, between my back and the fact that I'm soooo not 30 anymore. John and I used to joke and lament about the things we can't do because of aging bodies. The conversations, the laughter, the just being together. Gone. Bright in memory, and not the same thing.

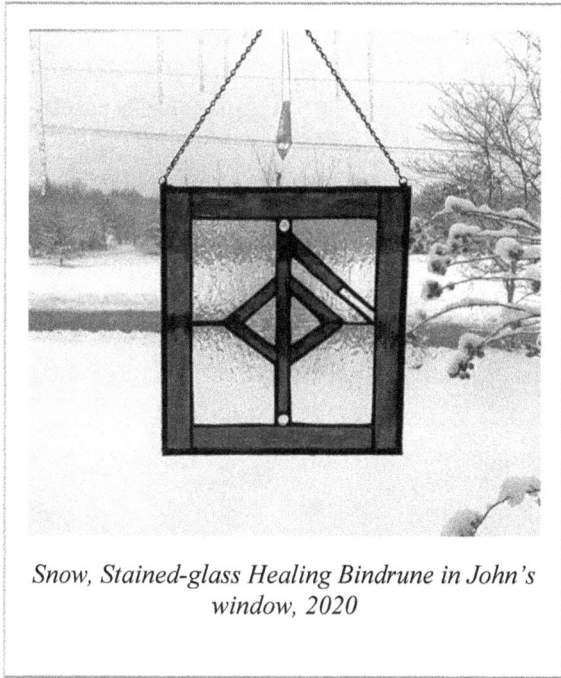

Snow, Stained-glass Healing Bindrune in John's window, 2020

This was one of John's favorite views, spring, summer, fall, winter.

The rage I wrote of in November just went away.

Apparently just getting it out there was the point.

Tuesday, February 16, 2021

Today is John's 71st birthday. It's been a hard day, very hard. A year ago it was almost 5 months since his death day and, looking back, I was still numb and in shock. This year? Not so much.

I miss you, John. I know you're near and it's not the same as your physical presence. I love you.

I took this photo in Lewes in November of 2010, shortly after we'd met. It's one of my favorite pictures of you.

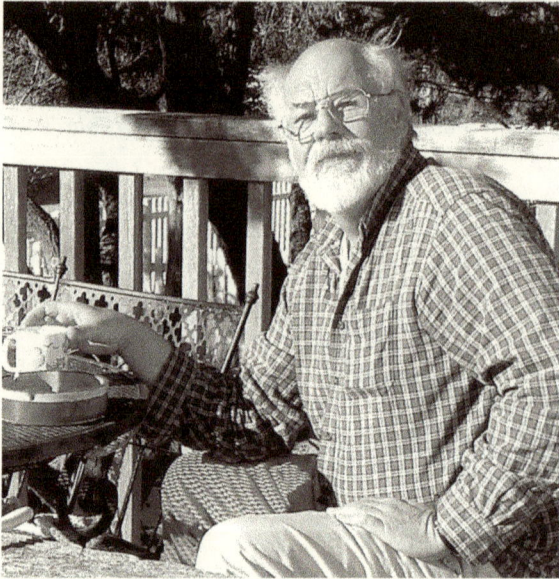

John in Lewes DE, November, 2010

I posted this on my public FB page and received some wonderful and thoughtful responses. Here are a few:

CC: He was one in a million!
CA: I lie here remembering his laughs. From the trials and
tribulations of life. The ups and downs of my life have taught me

that life is a blessing in the many forms it comes in. From sailing across the bay, to celebrating our first family cruise, my dad was always a man who always loved the earth and the beauty found in nature. May the seasons change and our love for my father forever dwell.

Cathi: *Love and more... .your photo captures his essence. "Preserve your memories..."* 💚

MG: *We all miss John. Take care*

ML: *Oh hon, I miss him too, and I miss you. Ugh, this year... Please let me know if I can support in any way*

NL: *Those days are hard. It's still "soon."*

RC: *from long years of loving and losing I can tell you how I understand. I think it takes at least three years to learn how to begin to manage such grief. I have loved and lost so many times. I have come to the conclusion which is true but not comforting. Life is about Losing.*

PS: *I remember John's dad very fondly. He loved to play bridge.*

Kerrith: *Love to you Elmdea – always.*

CS: *Sending love and hugs! He looks like a deeply good person.*

LJ: *Ya know it is weird the "whens" and "hows" of grief. The past few months have been the hardest ever. Yet it has been two years!*

DW: *I'm sure he has plenty to tell you upon the wind. Such love never dies.*

Bev: *As I have mentioned to you before, although I lost touch with John, much to my regret, it is comforting to feel that John finally met and spent cherished time with his soul mate. That must have been a great comfort to you both.*

LB: *May he live on in many hearts*

SA: *He looks wise and kind. Wish I could have met him.*

Joyce: *This IS a great picture of him*

Susan: *I hope each day gets better for you*

RR: *Hello John.*

Ed: *Thank you for sharing this. I'll share it with my family if it's okay.*

Elmdea: yes, it's very much ok.

KS: It can be a torturous, unending process. But it does get better eventually, I promise.

LR: Sending you warm hugs, Elmdea. I didn't know... I'm so sorry for your loss.

PB: Words may fall short or measure up to the moment to express what is deep within us ALL. It is with a Humble Witnessing, I acknowledge your grief, coupled with deep inner reflection. My Heart and Soul feels you

AS: I thought of him... what a nice photo, he looks so happy... I hope you are well, and once we are free of masks we can see each other! all the best!

Saturday, March 13, 2021

Second jab done as of 9 this morning. This time, the National Guard was helping with traffic. Again, a smooth and effortless experience and a whole lot of happy folks, me included. And yes, I'll continue to mask, distance, wash my hands cuz it makes sense.

I'm soooo relieved.

WV has done a super job! Today's vax site was a middle school gym. Totally works.

It really helps that I'm in a state that has a really good state-wide appointment system, one of the few.

Our vax cards are pink! I'm not sure why. I've only seen white ones shared here on FB, Moderna and Pfizer. It appears our county/health dept is an outlier with the pink. I likes it!

Tuesday, March 23, 2021

As of today, I've lived longer than John did. I'm not sure why it was important to me. I counted it out sometime in the early days of my grief, so I would know the day. So much counting of hours, days, weeks, months. From here on, I'll be older than John got to be.

Friday, May 7, 2021

I'm pleased and honored to let y'all know that my short story, *Hellbender Metamorphosis*, is one of 15 in *Particular Passages*, a new anthology that includes stories from many of my writing friends. This story is dear to my heart and tells of a lone Hellbender trying to save the last of his eggs from an increasingly polluted stream.

It's listed on multiple on-line stores (and purchases will make many people happy).

Wednesday, May 12, 2021

I am touched and inspired by a clarinetist's plans to play with the cicadas. There was an article in the NYT about this. Yet another way of connecting with the earth and its inhabitants. The 17 year Brood X cicadas will be singing quite loudly around here soon.

I'm still taking my daily walks and watching the small changes each day has been a gift. The slight growth of the grasses, the leaves out, the scents of early flowers (including the sassafras). And conversations with John as I walk.

Tuesday, May 18, 2021

Particular Passages has been out for two weeks now, after a bit of a rocky road getting it distributed to retailers. It should now be available through most any retailer you would like to purchase it from. Here's the Universal Link for it: *https://books2read.com/u/bx1vwv*

Friday, May 21, 2021

Today… today is our 10th wedding anniversary. We had 8 years and 4 months together and he's been gone a year and 8 months. This anniversary is a hard one for me. I'd been doing well, finding many days of peace and finding glimmers of who I am now.

I sense him around me at times and definitely last evening and this morning. Later this afternoon, I'll order take-out from the restaurant we usually went to for our anniversary: his favorite crab cakes and some crabby fries. I'll set a place for him at our table. I'll grieve, I'll remember, grateful we had the gift of the years we did, mourning the ones we no longer have together. I love you, John.

This picture is from our wedding, just after John had fed me a piece of wedding cake. We had sooo much fun!!!

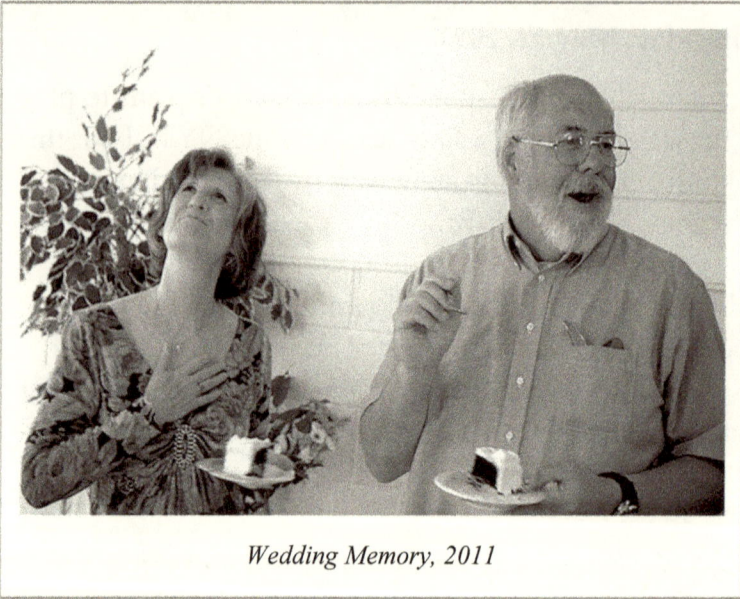

Wedding Memory, 2011

The responses from all of you today on social media have touched me. My heart has welcomed the peace and comfort you've sent. It has helped me navigate our anniversary and these following days. Such a journey grief is.

Sunday, July 25, 2021

Here I sit, wrapped up in your flannel shirt with the quilted lining, hugging myself. It's way too big and I don't care. It's the nearest I can come to a hug from you anymore. It's been 22 months since you died. I cry with the missing. Vaguely, I can feel you here. It helps.

Just yesterday, I discovered a new grief, a grief for the sweet memories, the good ones, the ordinary ones. It's taken me five months to figure out what this feeling in my chest is, that has raised my blood pressure and my anxiety. Tears finally came. I've been numb. Pandemic isolation means I haven't been able to be with those who really knew you, to cry together and hug each other. So I've become a bit numb, because that's what I knew to do given the shut-down state of the world.

Over the past three years, I've written so much about your illness and my grief, mostly for myself or a select group of friends on Facebook. It's time to read it and sort it out. I've been getting messages from Spirit that this would be a good thing. I didn't want to listen.

I'm tired, in body and in soul. May this prove helpful.

Saturday, August 21, 2021

Today, I put away most of the pillows on the couch. There were too many and it was too much work to get them off if I wanted to lie down for a quick nap.

Now I understand why I had to pull them out of storage and put them on the couch. I thought it was because I wanted to see and use them again, to begin making small changes in the house. I was making a change, but not the one I thought I was.

As I look at the couch tonight, it looks bare. The memories of John lying on it for months during the day are more present. I can almost see him there. He'd go upstairs in the evenings, but spend most of the day on the couch. Then he couldn't manage the stairs anymore and slept on the couch. It was too short for him, and he did it anyway.

The memory of him, lying on the couch. It's alive for me as it hasn't been for almost two years.

Tuesday, August 24, 2021

I've started putting together the timeline for this book.

I'm going through John's Medical Notebook that I put together shortly after he was diagnosed. There are notes in here that I don't remember. Mostly, in the moment, I'm feeling something that feels like relief. I'm far enough away from those days that I can see the bigger picture. I'm not teary, feeling grief. What will be interesting is to see how I do later today/tonight, what feelings come up.

* * *

There is a tightness in my throat. Yes, now I'm feeling the slight tightness in my chest and the beginnings of tears. So much neither of us realized at the time. So much I didn't realize at the time. I don't think I could afford to. I was in John survival mode and me survival mode.

I've just been looking at late June/early July of 2019, when we shifted from cancer treatment to Hospice. Reading what I'd written about his declining ability to communicate and how much it wore him out. Chemo killed him faster than the cancer would have. I absolutely believe that.

Thursday, August 26, 2021

I've made it through most of the notebook. There are times when it's felt like I was living it again, that John was alive and here. I've cried, experiencing at a distance the suffering of both of us. It's so clear.

I don't think I could fully feel it at the time. I needed my energy and focus to be on John and making sure things were as good as was possible for him. All the appointments, driving here and there, advocating for him and with him for himself took more energy and focus than I realized at the time. It was a horror show of suffering, with increasing awareness that only death would end it.

I'm crying as I write this, my chest and throat tight. Paradoxically, I'm experiencing relief. I've been afraid of revisiting this for nearly two years. It isn't as hard or as painful as I'd feared.

These almost two years since John died have allowed me to remember more of the times before he began to be sick, without them being overshadowed by the seven horrible months of painful physical, mental, and emotional decline he experienced as he was dying.

I need to do something to care for myself. Knitting is what comes to mind. It requires a certain amount of focus and the repetition is calming.

Sunday, August 29, 2021

Today, Hurricane Ida struck New Orleans and the Louisiana / Mississippi coasts. The same date Hurricane Katrina hit in 2005, 16 years ago.

I'm struck by my personal response to Ida compared to Katrina. Katrina sent my then unidentified catastrophizing self into major action. I call that part of me Miz C (for Miz Catastrophizer). I watched in dismay as the federal government sent so little help. A major belief system was destroyed during those days. A belief that the federal government was there to help in major disasters. It wasn't.

I went over the top in my response. I drew up lists of old crafts that needed to be learned by people. I researched the minimum number of people who would be needed in a group to survive (eight, though twenty would be better). I went survivalist / prepper, despite the fact that nothing in my life had changed. But I was seeing disaster all around me and couldn't understand why others weren't. My formerly safe world wasn't anymore. In retrospect, I had been blind to what had been going on, politically and environmentally. I wasn't after that.

With Hurricane Ida, I've been grateful to see federal help

sent in before and after the storm. There's so much else going on that much of that is being overshadowed.

Miz C is behaving herself. I'm grateful.

I'm sad my expectations are so low. Perhaps that's realism. Perhaps that's wisdom. I'm unsure it matters much. What I know for certain is, despite the challenges and griefs, I've had a blessed life. I've always had shelter, food, clothing, friends. Always. I acknowledge my privilege. I share when and as appropriate, in my own community, in small ways. I don't need to be seen.

John and I knew that there would be hard times coming. I always thought we'd meet them together. We still are, but he's over there and I'm here. It isn't the same.

Friday, September 3, 2021

I took last night's roasted Costco chicken out of the fridge, ready to cut it up some more and heat it up for dinner. I'm looking at it. It strikes me that, when John was alive, we would have eaten about half of it for the first meal. Alone, I'll get four, maybe five meals from it. And the tears came. A grief burst. I had to sit down and just let myself cry. It was only a minute or so and I so miss him. I could almost feel him sitting at his usual place at the dinner table. Almost. It will never be anything more than "almost".

It's seventeen days until September 20, the second deathiversary. Anniversary isn't the right word. That sounds like a celebration. I confess to a bit of dread, wondering if I'll be hit with anxiety, verging on panic, like I was in February or in May. I'll find out. I've learned how to manage them better… and still.

The heaviness is rising in my chest, tears coming to my eyes as I write this. Grief doesn't go away. It shifts and changes. It doesn't leave. It's not present in every moment. I don't wake up to it and I rarely go to sleep with it. But it does rise up.

Grief burst is the best description. Like a rain burst.

Sunday, September 5, 2021

It's eye-opening, going through the FB posts and journals of those months of caregiving. Both easier and harder than I'd thought. Easier because time has softened the memories of those last seven months, so filled with grief and sorrow and the unknown. Harder because I can see now what I couldn't / wouldn't see then: the steady, unrelenting progress of John's cancer. While I'm seeing some things I would have liked to change, I couldn't then because I didn't know then what I knew later or now.

What strikes me this morning is my focus after John died: that his death and dying had broken me open and I wasn't going to ignore that last gift from him. I was determined to learn and grow. I called and call it a "gift" because it's the only word I can find that comes close to honoring our experience together as he was dying and after he died. I've no idea how, or even if, other grievers have this same feeling. I just know it's mine.

I've done inner work my whole life. There's been no reason to change that. I'm in several grief groups on social media and a number of people have ranted about how much they hate (literally *hate*, whew!) the whole growing through / with your grief. I get that.

But it gave me a purpose. I was still alive for a reason. I needed (and still need) to believe that to keep myself going. It gives me a reason to get up each day, feed myself, and attempt to figure out how to live in social isolation because of Covid-19. I've grown and I've changed. The essential me is still here. But the outside bits have shifted. There are days when I'd just as soon die and join John. I'm not suicidal, but I'd rather just not be here. I know other grievers get this. This world is beautiful and ugly, gentle and brutal. I'd like a rest.

On another note, Miz Alice, who was John's cat, has taken to napping on the 2' x 3' green rug that used to be in front of his chair on the smoking porch. I moved it a week or so ago to in front of the front door. She's never napped in front of the door before. It's completely new behavior.

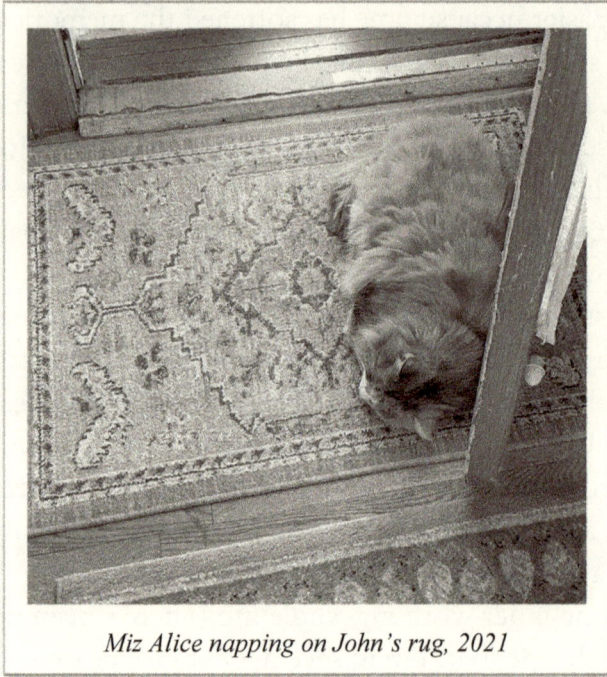

Miz Alice napping on John's rug, 2021

When John was ill, he wanted as much green around him as possible. It felt healing for him. I got that little rug for in front of his chair on the smoking porch. We kept the door to that porch closed so the house didn't smell like smoke. That rug stayed on that porch until a few weeks ago when, in an on-line auction, I won a runner that fits the front hallway. I realized that small rug went well with the new-to-me runner, so I swapped out the black one that had been there since I first met John.

Alice has been sleeping on it for hours and hours every day since then. She never laid on the black one. I wonder if there's still some faint John scent there? Or John energy? I'll never know. She was John's cat. He was the one she came to at the shelter, sick and weak as she was. I suspect that she, too, is grieving still and lying on this rug is her getting as close to him as she can. Part of me envies her.

* * *

I just re-read this from my June 30, 2019 journal entry:

> *"I suspect the grief will feel somewhat like I felt after Mouse and Zinnia died – intense for a bit, then dwindling. I'll always be missing him."*

I soooooo had no clue!! At almost the second anniversary of John's death, grief is still quite present. Not sharp like it was. But very much here. It's not going anywhere because this IS where it lives, rightfully and properly, here in my heart.

Tuesday, September 7, 2021

Miz Alice is still sleeping on the small rug that used to be under John's feet. She only moves if I need to go in or out the front door. Even the vacuum cleaner (which she isn't a fan of) doesn't move her away from that rug. I had no idea. I would have put it out much earlier if I'd known.

I'm in tears right now. For some reason, I thought I might listen to the recording I made February 15, 2019 at our first visit to the medical oncologist in Baltimore. Friends had suggested I record it so I could double check what I remembered. I haven't listened to it since maybe March of 2019. It lives on my phone but I've hardly thought of it over these past two years. Now I think I know why. I wasn't ready.

I have three short voicemails from John, but they don't really sound like him. He didn't like phones. They were a necessary evil, as far as he was concerned. His voice in this recording is the John voice I remember and recognize. I don't have a memory for voices, never have, with a few very rare exceptions. John hasn't been one of them. Hearing his voice brings back so many of our conversations. I miss him. I miss him.

Wednesday, September 8, 2021

I hadn't thought I'd be posting much here after John died. That's been mostly true, and there are some times when I feel called to. Today is one of those times.

It's twelve days until the second anniversary of John's physical death. I, who have trouble remembering the sounds of a voice in my head, now clearly remember the tone, cadence, and words of the few words of his I heard on the recording yesterday: "I am physically tired."

Lately I've been remembering there's a short part somewhere in that recording where John is talking about a bear wandering into the yard while he was outside, grilling dinner. The doctor and the intern were much taken aback, and John had to continue the tale, in the way he would when such opportunities arose.

As much as I think I'd like to hear that, I'm unsure I can handle listening to the recording to get there and then, once there, if I can handle hearing his so beloved voice in storytelling mode. No decision needs to be made today, or tomorrow, or… I'll know when / if it's time.

There are tears here somewhere. They start to surge up from my heart, my chest feels like it constricts, my throat tightens, and the tears evaporate before spilling from my eyes.

Grief comes in so many ways. I now suspect I'll always be learning its new shapes, forms, and subtleties. Today, I'm feeling stretched, as my being makes room for this new aspect of grief, the grief that all we were together here hasn't continued. It's stalled, stopped, because he's no longer here for us to continue to weave our lives together.

Yes, I know his spirit is always near. I'm grateful. And it isn't the same. It lacks touch, sound, the physical energy of a living presence.

His physical absence feels more real. It's felt real since he took his last breath. I guess it's just getting realer. I suspect it has to do with the length of time since 8:12 a.m., September 20, 2019. Some part of me has wanted to deny this truth of his physical absence from the world. Perhaps because I wasn't yet ready to hold and carry this next aspect of grief.

Like all previous anniversaries (death, birthdays, marriage, day of diagnosis, holidays), the days and weeks leading up to this one are becoming difficult, the grief more raw and present. I'll know in twelve days if the actual anniversary day is easier. It has been in the past, but things change.

The prospect of another winter of relative, but hopefully not total, isolation isn't helping. I've more tools to deal with that, but it's still very hard.

Thank you for being my witnesses. I'm so very grateful to all of you in my life. Knowing you are all here, living, being, growing, helps immensely.

Thursday, September 9, 2021

I had expected that I'd get fewer reactions and responses to yesterday's post. It makes absolute sense to me. It's almost two years out. Culturally, we're expected to have "moved on" after six or so months. Nope.

I'm in a number of grief groups and again and again, what comes up is how thoughtless people are, how triggering, how forgetful friends, family, and co-workers are of the most important date in the poster's life, especially the death date. These posts are usually from people in their second plus year of grief.

I get it. Before John died, I thought I understood grief. A number of people, including my father, had died and grief didn't last all that long. It was there for a while, a few months, max. What I didn't and couldn't understand was that the depth of grief depends entirely on the depth of the relationship. I now "get it."

I'm the only one with me day in and day out. The anniversaries, of whatever kind, are mine. Very few are shared with anyone else. Yes, my sister and I know each other's birthdays and our mother's birthday. Other important dates? Not so much.

Paradoxically, because of the lack of comments on my post, a space has opened up inside me. I, and I alone, am responsible for how I move forward from here. There is something spacious in that understanding. It's always been true that I'm responsible for how I meet my life, but it feels more true now. There is more room for me to move forward, to meet new people, to be an elder. There is much I still don't know or understand. I'm increasingly comfortable with that.

Wednesday, September 15, 2021

I've just finished going through my writing from March, 2019. What strikes me now is how fast John's health spiraled out and down. In a matter of 3 weeks, while weak, he went from being alert and mostly awake during the day, to constant nausea, thrush, and cellulitis that verged on sepsis.

At the time, it didn't seem that fast. I was just doing the next thing and the next thing and trying to keep myself together. My meltdown on March 20 makes even more sense now. Without the support of my friends, I'm not sure I'd have done as well as I did.

Monday, September 20, 2021

I began today much as I do these days: got up, washed up and dressed, sat in meditation, fixed my morning smoothie, and then went for a walk. When I got back, it was near the time John had died two years ago. I got out the beeswax 24-

hour Yahrzeit Candle and lit it. I placed it in front of a picture of him taken shortly after we met, back in August of 2010. Beside it I placed the statue of Columbia, to honor his work as a prosecutor and then as a public defender. Kuan Yin was on the other side, the goddess of great compassion. I placed his small statues of Freya and Skadi, two of his favorite Norse goddesses, on either side of the candle, with the small urn of his ashes in front of the candle. I placed his watch, then lit a stick of his favorite incense: Dragon's Blood. Quite eclectic from a spiritual perspective, and it worked for me.

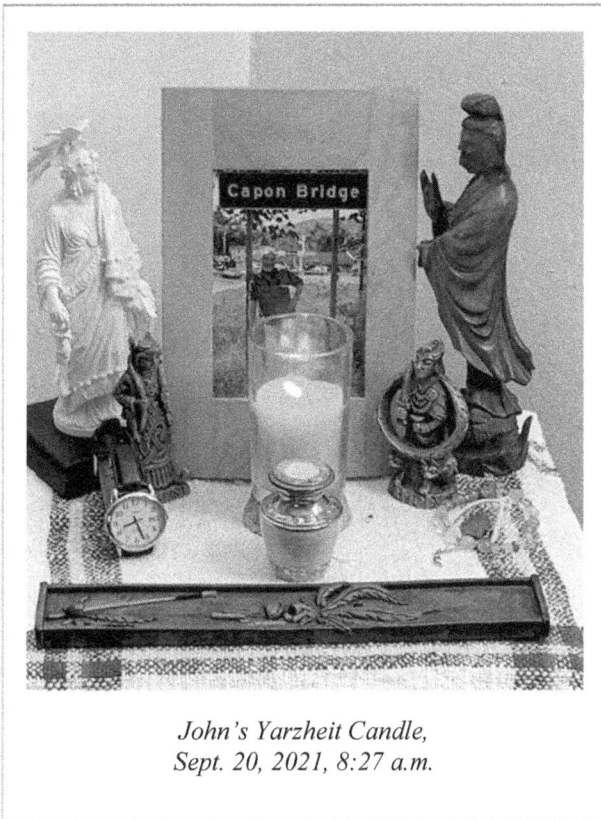

John's Yarzheit Candle,
Sept. 20, 2021, 8:27 a.m.

Cathi introduced me to Yahrzeit last year, on the one year anniversary of John's death. Yahrzeit is a Yiddish word meaning the commemoration of the death of a loved one on the anniversary of their death. I found some Yahrzeit candles on Amazon, and ordered two of them in April. At this point, I'm glad I remembered I had them. Grief brain still shows up, combined with the whole pandemic brain thing.

A few weeks back, I'd asked Margi if we could do a small ceremony of some sort at Stillpoint, an octagonal building on her family property that has been used for small ceremonies and rituals for many years. It was built with much love by her mother and local friends.

Last night, I gathered a number of things together: John's picture, his wallet, a small bird statue he'd had on his personal altar, a mini urn of his ashes, his still-running watch, a seashell, a smudge stick, a bird wing to fan the smudge, a rattle. This morning, I realized today's ceremony wasn't about John. It was about and for me as I continue to move forward with my life, continuing to carry my grief as a companion I'm getting to know better and better without being overwhelmed. I took his mini urn, the small candle that burned when his body was blessed after his death, and a lighter.

Margi and I walked the short woodland path to Stillpoint, admiring the wide variety of mushrooms that have popped up. We entered the building and I could feel the peace, like a soft blanket, enfolding me.

We sat and Margi called the directions. We spoke of grief, of learning, of growing. I then shared the sounds I heard last night. I'd gone to bed, window open, when a blood curdling death shriek came from the field across the road. There may have been a faint owl hoot when the shriek stopped. "Rabbit, caught by an owl." was my thought. "Poor rabbit." Followed by "Owls gotta eat." Margi mentioned that foxes also have a pretty spine shivering call that sounds like something in extreme pain. I wanted to meditate on its meaning, so we did.

Sitting in the silence, breathing, mind slowing. "It's what

life is here on this planet. It doesn't matter if it was a rabbit, a fox, or another animal. Life and death are what happens here." I "felt" John hug me, as though he was sitting behind me, and my meditation was done.

As we were finishing up, Margi asked if I'd been aware of when the wind chimes rang. "No. I remember hearing them, faintly, but that's all."

"They only chimed twice, once when I was speaking about John and again when you were sharing that John had hugged you during your meditation. It's windy out and normally they would be chiming more."

I smiled as I took a short, deep breath. "Ah. Yes, I know he's around, I'm just not always aware of it. Thank you."

As we walked back up the woodland path, Margi stopped and picked up a stone. "Here, this is for you."

She put it in my hand. A squarish stone, half red stone of some sort and half quartz, with a crack in it with a small piece of green moss. Holding it, looking at it, it's a physical representation of this world and the next, of love and grief, and life that insists on being. It sits on my small home altar now.

When I returned home, the driveway was being finished. It was fascinating to watch, how they knew just how much depth of loose asphalt to spread so that, when they ran the vibrating roller over it, it would match the height of the asphalt they'd laid yesterday. It was all finished, equipment gone, by about 4.

Over the course of the day, I would sit at my dining room table, looking at the Yahrzeit candle, remembering, as I gazed at the flame and his picture. It was good.

Cathi let me know she'd lit one for John, too. She shared that her grandmother used to say "if the candle burns longer than 24 hours, you can be sure the spirit of your lost departed lives on".

I lit John's Yahrzeit Candle at 8:27 a.m. on September 20, 2021; it was still burning the following morning. It went out around 9:25 a.m., September 21, 2021, almost a full 25 hours after I lit it.

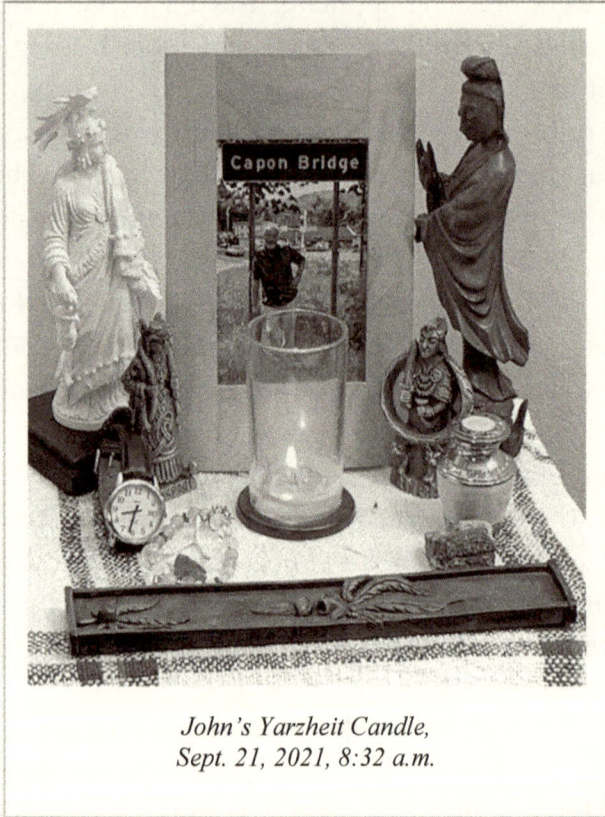

John's Yarzheit Candle,
Sept. 21, 2021, 8:32 a.m.

Looking Back

Year two of grieving was about coming to terms with the reality and finality of John's physical death. The first year was about making it through all the firsts: so, so many of them. I had no plan for the second year. There were still a few firsts, all related to house and property maintenance, which now fell to me.

I often wonder how different year two might have been without the pandemic, and if I had been able to get together with John's family and friends, so we could mourn together. I'll never know.

That year, I found a private FB group for those of us who had lost our partners or children. I lurked more than I posted, but reading of everyone else's experiences helped me feel less alone and realize how normal my grief experience is. It was comforting to know that some had to keep their beloved's closet exactly as it had been, while others, like myself, had to let go of as much as possible soon after their beloved's death. Both are valid. It's so very individual.

We all grieve in our own, unique way. And those of us who have known deep, catastrophic grief know and understand each other. We know our experiences aren't identical, but the core foundations of our grief are the same

PART XII:
YEAR THREE

Tuesday, September 22, 2021

The driveway was finished yesterday, before the heavy rains predicted for last night into this evening. It's so odd, looking at it. Foreign. It's what I've wanted and it's no longer what it was when John was alive. Like so much since John died.

Sitting in meditation this morning, my mind and emotions wouldn't settle. Year Two is complete. It's now Year Three. Such a long time and no time at all. That phrase feels more real to me than it ever has. Time does march on and it feels harder, less kind now, in some odd way, since John died.

It makes sense. He's not here and the more time passes, the further away he becomes in my lived, everyday experience. He becomes more and more memory and less and less reality. Reality is this life here, alone, taking care of feeding myself, going shopping, taking care of the property, looking after Miz Alice. Building a dream and hope in the form of a teardrop trailer and the possibility of going to small gatherings of friends without worrying about Covid.

What I'm feeling is melancholy: a sad missing for what was and won't be again, mixed with gratitude for my house and the ease of my life. There's also the reassurance of having a fair idea how this Year Three will be: many periods of time purely focused on here and now, interspersed with grief bursts which will often take me by surprise. The anniversaries will come, be experienced, and moved beyond. Time is constant, both relentless and reassuring.

Texting with Cathi yesterday, I'd shared that the driveway was being paved and that it was pure synchronicity it was happening over the second anniversary of John's death, since I'd contracted for it back in early May and asphalt supply for non-road projects was sometimes iffy.

"For me," I wrote, "it represents loving forward and new pathways that will reveal themselves as they will."

Except what I was thinking was *"living forward."* My fingers and my heart knew better.

John's death did break me open. I grieve, sometimes deeply, sometimes in a passing thought, and every grief in between. That will continue for the rest of my life. There may be more time between grief bursts… or not. I've been blessed with experiencing great love. John's watch continues to tick on. At some point, like him, it will stop. My assumption is I'll continue on after that.

I'm at peace in this moment, making friends with melancholy, a new aspect of my grief.

Sunday, September 26, 2021

I'm still trying to get used to the new driveway. I've been looking at old pictures of it. It was my friendly, known driveway, even if I wasn't real happy with the summer mud puddles and the snow plow moving the gravel all over the place.

I realized this afternoon that some part of me wants the paved driveway gone. I want it back the way it was. I miss it. Never mind that I've been looking forward to having it paved, having a real driveway instead of a half grass/half gravel car path.

Digging into that a bit more, I think it's because it's a major home improvement, with no input from John. We'd never talked about paving it. I almost can't look at it. It feels silly to feel that way combined with… ah, yes… mourning the passing of yet another aspect of our shared lives. This driveway is me committing to greater comfort in this house for however many years I continue to live here.

It's quite clear to me that grief is still here. Intellectually, I know that's reasonable. Emotionally, I know that, too. And some part of me wants it done, complete, gone, back to the old me. That old me isn't here anymore. She was the foundation for the current me. It's always been this way.

I'm just rattling away here, trying to find some clarity. I think I need to move and breathe, take a walk, knit, weave, something to occupy my mind other than this continuing life without John. I'm just missing him a lot today. It is what it is. And here I thought, waaaaay back when, that grief would be like my grief for my two cats. Such innocence.

This grief isn't as intense as it was while John was sick and dying, or after he died. It doesn't occupy the whole of my days. It doesn't cut as deep. Instead, it rests heavy in my chest. I'll cry, it will lighten, but it never goes away.

If I was given the choice between loving and grieving John or never having met and loved him, I'll still take loving and grieving.

Wednesday, February 16, 2022

Today is John's 72nd birthday. He's been gone for 2 years and almost 5 months now. I continue to grieve for him, though it's softer now than it was in the beginning. My memories of our years together are now what I remember most, rather than the last 10 months when he was so ill and dying. I'm grateful. He's "visited" me a number of times over these past years. It's a great comfort to me. The picture here is my current favorite of him, taken in Lewes, DE in late 2010, several months after we first met.

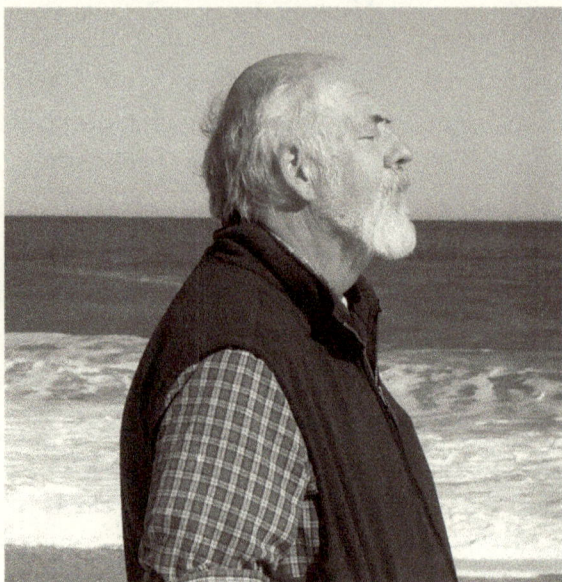

John in Lewes DE,
Nov, 2010

As well as my grief for John, I'm in anticipatory grief for my 94 year old mother. She's in hospice at her continuous care facility. Last week I was in Phoenix to say my in-person goodbyes. I got to hold her hand, give and receive hugs, bring her bundt-inis (the most amazing mini bundt cakes!), and we both resolved the on again/off again issues we've had with each other. I feel great peace and love. And grief. She's the only person I've known my whole life. I can't imagine the world without her in it. And I'll soon be living in that world.

This evening, the auction of all her household goods, her weaving, her weaving notes, her "things" will end. It's another kind of goodbye. Sooooo many memories tied to so much of it. While my sister and I took a few things, most of them are going. We don't have room for them and are doing our own cleaning out of "stuff." We sent some to her brother, to her grandson, and to a friend. This picture of her is from 2010 when we moved her into the apartment that is now being cleared out.

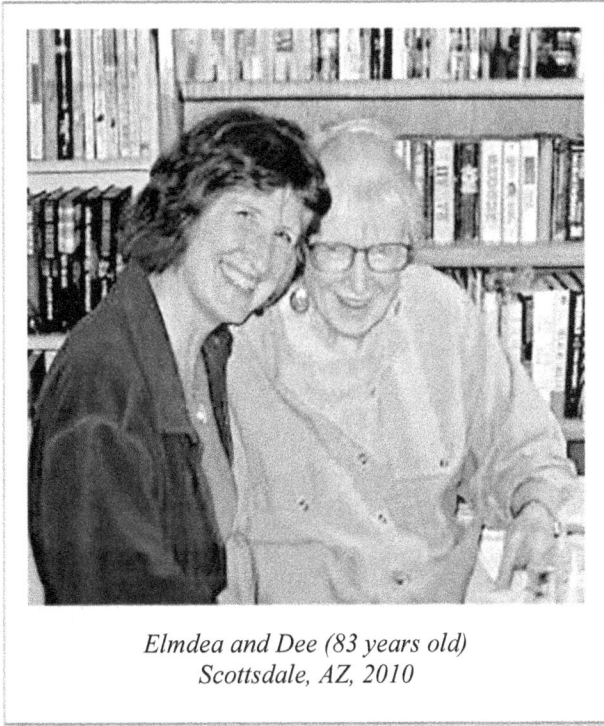

Elmdea and Dee (83 years old)
Scottsdale, AZ, 2010

Sunday, April 3, 2022

It's a little over two and half years since John's death. Two years into the pandemic and the isolation. I'm vaxed and boosted, I'm getting out more, and I'm still alone. John's not here. He's still the only one I really want to be with, talk with, interact with. He's still not here.

This morning I lost it, crying harder and deeper than I have in quite awhile. I had to give Miz Alice her pain meds for an ear infection and swollen ear. The meds are liquid, pre-loaded into a little syringe. She wasn't being at all helpful, not that she has been. She is a cat, after all. John's cat. She's been sleeping on his bed this whole time she's been sick. I'm guessing her sensitive nose can smell him still and she finds comfort in that. I wish my nose was.

I burst into tears, frustrated and overwhelmed. I pleaded with her to help me, it was for her own good and comfort. I finally wrapped her up in a towel and squirted it into her mouth, sobbing the whole time.

I recognized the feeling. That feeling of helplessness when John was in Hospice and we knew he was dying, slowly but surely. Knowing there was only so much I could do. Knowing that no matter how hard I wanted, I couldn't do anything to make it all go away and be better. The only physical thing I could do was make sure there were always enough pain and nausea meds. Friends kept telling me that just being there for him was enough. It never felt like enough. I didn't have, and I still don't have, a magic wand.

I'm writing this hours later and I'm still crying, not as hard. It's another level of the missing and the knowing he'll never be back, not physically. When he was here, he gave Miz Alice any meds she needed and there wasn't any fight or resistance on her part.

So many things were so much easier when John was here. I wasn't alone, I was loved just as I was. I didn't have to make all the decisions by myself. We talked about them. He'd remind me to eat when I'd forget, or to call my oldest friend, Susan. Or so many other things. Just as I did for him when he would hit something emotional or hard. We did that for each other.

I'm so tired of doing it alone… again. Yes, having lived a little less than half my adult life as a single female in this society has helped. It's still hard.

I've been grieving him more at this two and half year mark than I have been for months. A deeper layer of it. My grief for John is now part of me. I'd actually miss it if it went away.

While mornings like this are really, really hard, I'll still take this over never having known and loved him, and been loved by him.

And so it is. My life continues, carrying my love and missing. The pain isn't as searing as it was. It's part of me now, instead of something life imposed on me. There will be new awarenesses, deeper levels of grief, and I'll still breathe, fix meals, enjoy beautiful days, explore new things, laugh, live, until my time here is done and I can leave this body and join him on the other side.

I know I'm repeating myself here. That I've written this before. And I need the reminding, the comparisons, so see how much has changed and how much hasn't.

Wednesday, April 20, 2022

It all started innocently enough. My computer was doing some weird stuff, so I figured it needed a tune-up. Its last one was probably four years ago, when John did it.

The computer guy got here Monday and I asked whether it made sense to keep my computer or switch to John's. After some checking, he said mine has more memory. However, he said he could get a few hundred dollars for John's. Okay. But I want it all backed up on an external hard drive. No problem, he said.

Today, he brought my computer back and got everything connected. He said it was virus free and just needed the dust removed. He also took the big BENQ monitor that John had. Turns out it was/is an expensive gaming monitor. It was too big for me.

What has taken me by surprise is the sense of loss I'm feeling. It makes sense, now that I think about it. John and his computer, his on-line gaming, were core parts of who he was. His computer and his monitor are gone. The desk looks eerily blank, stark, strange.

It's no accident that today, the two year and seven month anniversary of John's death, is now also the date when his gaming computer and monitor have left, to find their new homes. It really didn't make any sense for them to just be sitting here, unused. But they were part of John, part of his identity, a big part of his life. One more piece gone.

Sunday, May 8, 2022

I did a three-way FaceTime with Dee (my mother – our parents had us call them by their given names) and Becky (my sister). Dee told me I'm beautiful and said, "you're a good one." What a beautiful blessing.

Her face. Her face is soooo peaceful, with a quiet joy. It's not something I've seen there before. I gently blew her a kiss over the phone. Perhaps thirty seconds later, she brought her hand up to the side of her face, slowly, as if receiving the kiss.

Earlier, Becky had asked if she was scared. "No, I'm ready to go home."

This is such a huge change. All my life, Dee has insisted that mind and brain are one and the same and, when we die, that's it. There's nothing after that, no memories, no "other" life, nothing. That death is a final and total wiping out of all personal consciousness. She couldn't envision, let alone accept, the concept of "going home" to something after death. My sense of it is she's been walking between the worlds quite a bit of late.

Wednesday, May 11, 2022

Today I flew out to Phoenix. I just have to be there. I'm planning on staying a week, since I have appointments I need to keep back home. No, Dee isn't actively dying, but Becky needs support. I know what grief is, now. I didn't before. I want to be there for her.

We went straight from the airport to the Health Center. There's no way I was going to fly out here and not see her and then have her die tonight. Not happening.

Friday, May 13, 2022

Today, Becky and I told Dee that it was OK for her to go. She was asleep when we told her, but she woke up briefly and smiled, such a sweet smile, peaceful, with that same quiet joy.

Not long after that, I was reaching for something behind her Bose radio on top of her dresser and it turned on. I hadn't touched it and the remote was in a bag on her bedside table. Becky and I looked at each other, kind of spooked. I turned and looked at the Bose, front and back, top, sides. There weren't any buttons and touching it didn't turn it off. We can only assume someone (spirit) decided she needed classical music playing.

Saturday, May 14, 2022

I re-checked the Bose today. If I touch it just towards the front of the top, it turns off and on. Except yesterday, I'd maybe touched it near the back.

Dee told us that she had a lot of books and someone was giving a talk. She was quite happy and wanted to go back to the talk. She went back to sleep.

This reminds me of some descriptions I've read about different places of gathering and learning on the other side and how much fun and how exciting they are. I suspect she's already visiting them.

Sunday, May 15, 2022

Dee was very lucid today! It felt like what I've heard described as a rally. Becky and I again told her it was OK for her to leave. I stood behind Becky, my arms around her, as we told Dee we were and will be taking care of each other. She doesn't need to worry about us.

She asked for her pillows, the one's she'd woven. I watched her right hand as her fingers touched that weaving, like they (and she) were remembering the weaving and the making. She was such a gifted weaver, with a sure eye for color combinations. She worked hard at it, starting in her 50's, creating many beautiful things.

Her hands. Something about her hands seems so precious right now.

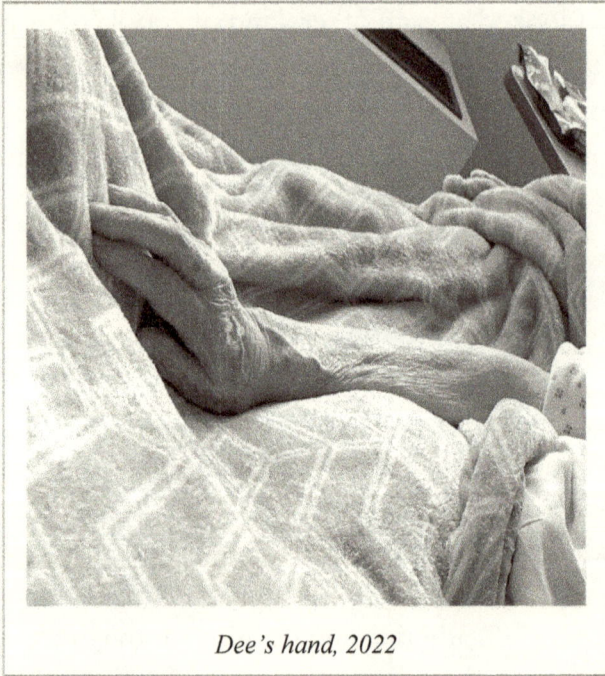

Dee's hand, 2022

Monday, May 16, 2022

Dee was deeply asleep today. She hasn't eaten all day and she's drunk very little, according to the nurses.

Wednesday, May 18, 2022

We were with Dee for about two hours. She was kinda here and kinda not. She still hasn't eaten anything and hasn't drunk much either. We aren't sure why she's still hanging on, but she is.

She was in some pain, so she was given more morphine.

I'm flying home on Saturday, the 21st. I'd wanted to be here so Becky and I could be together when and after Dee died. I don't think that's going to happen.

Thursday, May 19, 2022

Independently of each other, Becky and I decided I won't see Dee again before I leave. Becky will tell her I've flown home. Why? In case that's what she's waiting for. I had to check in with myself to make sure that was the right thing. When I imagined not seeing her, it felt comfortable and OK. When I imagined seeing her again, I realized it was all mental stuff. So telling her I've left is the right thing.

Saturday, May 21, 2022

I was supposed to fly home today but my flight was delayed and I wouldn't get home until after dark and I'm not driving in the dark. It doesn't work so well for me anymore. By the time I was able to call in to change flights, the earliest one that would get me home in the daytime leaves on Wednesday, the 24th, so I'm here a few more days.

Tuesday, May 23, 2022

Much to my surprise, Dee came to me during my morning meditation. I wasn't attempting to reach her, let alone expecting to hear from her. I'm sensing she's quite busy right now as she prepares to leave her body and this world, whenever that will be. She told me she's fine and she'll be in touch. That there's some work we will be doing together. Then she was gone.

It was a sense of her, rather than a visual. I'm now curious about what that will be. I didn't get the sense that it was about resolving anything, as we did that in February. This felt more like some project.

Sunday, May 28, 2022

When Becky and I talked last night, I asked her if she knew if the Health Center would call her as soon as they knew that Dee had died. She wasn't sure. I then told her I'd be keeping the phone by my bed from here on out.

Hospice called Becky at 4:04 a.m.. They'd been called earlier and came and confirmed Dee's death, filling out the appropriate paperwork. The nurse said that Dee had died around 2:30 a.m., as they check on those who are close to death more frequently. I remember that from when John died and how the reported time of death was different from the actual time of death.

Becky called me three minutes later, after she got off the phone with hospice.

I'm kind of in shock, close to tears, but not. She's gone.

Saturday, June 4, 2022

January 30, 1928 to May 28, 2022 are the dates that bracket my mother's life. It's now a week since she died. It still feels unreal, and quite right at the same time. She was 94. Her body was failing, she couldn't walk, she was tired physically and emotionally. She was ready, more than ready, to rest and to leave.

She left a legacy of intellectual curiosity; a love of learning; beautiful weaving; and love for her great-granddaughter, her grandson, her granddaughter-in-law, her daughters, and her younger brother.

She was a strong woman. In the 1950's and '60's, my father would leave on business for a week or so and leave her with no money for food or gas. He just didn't, for whatever reason. The money was surely there. He was a top scientist with the government. My mother learned to make one chicken feed us for at least four meals. I remember how determined she was in the early 1970's to make a life for herself. She became an LPN, divorced my father, learned to weave, and became a published and highly respected weaver. No small thing for that time.

She once told me that it was hard, growing up with the working women of WWII and Clare Booth Luce (writer, U.S. Ambassador, author) as role models and then, after the war, being told that all the jobs were for the returning veterans and the women were to get married and have babies. End of story.

What has surprised me, which surprises me, is how much of my mother is in me: my love of classical music, my love of books and reading, my appreciation of colors and their interactions, my love of southwest jewelry, and the list goes on.

I've cried some, but not lots. This grief is so different from my grief for John. That makes sense, since they were totally different relationships. This grief isn't as raw, as tearing at my soul. It feels gentler. I somehow just know that she's OK and she'll be in touch when it's time for whatever it is we'll be working on together. John helped me learn that this is true.

I'm pretty much wearing a ring of hers 24/7. It's silver and turquoise, the silver band worn down on one side.

The pictures: Dee in 1956, at 28; my grandmother, Dora, Dee (at 35), and me knitting in 1963; Dee, at 75 on the California coast (2003); and the two of us (Dee at 90), in her apartment (2018).

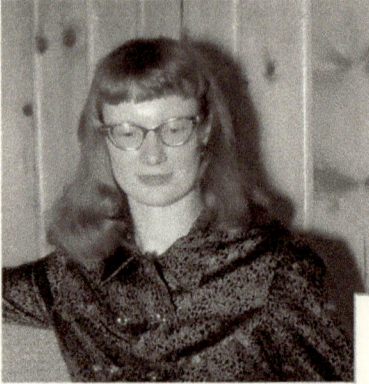

Dee at 28,
Boulder, CO (1956)

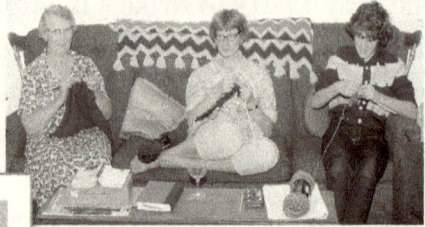

Dora, Dee (35), & Elmdea,
knitting on the couch,
Fort Collins, CO (1964)

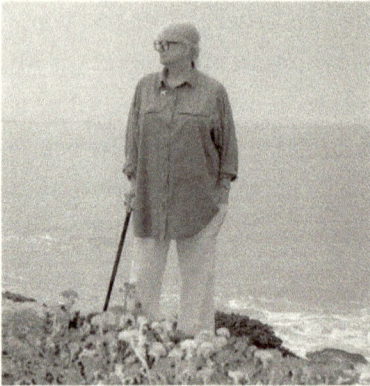

Dee at 75,
Cambria, CA (2003)

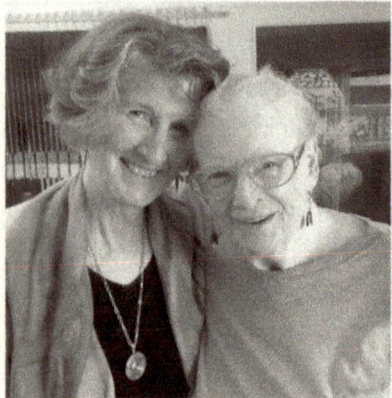

Elmdea and Dee (2018)

Wednesday, August 10, 2022

A Facebook friend, who lost her husband about the same time I lost John, recently wrote that her grief was going through a rough patch, a *"delayed, or protracted or stymied experience... because of Covid."* That rings true for me, too. The isolation, the limited sharing of memories with those who knew our beloved and now... less isolation but not much sharing.

Sunday, September 11, 2022

I had a vivid dream last night. It's stayed with me half the day, so I decided to make a collage. It's called "Hope." It's a welcome message.

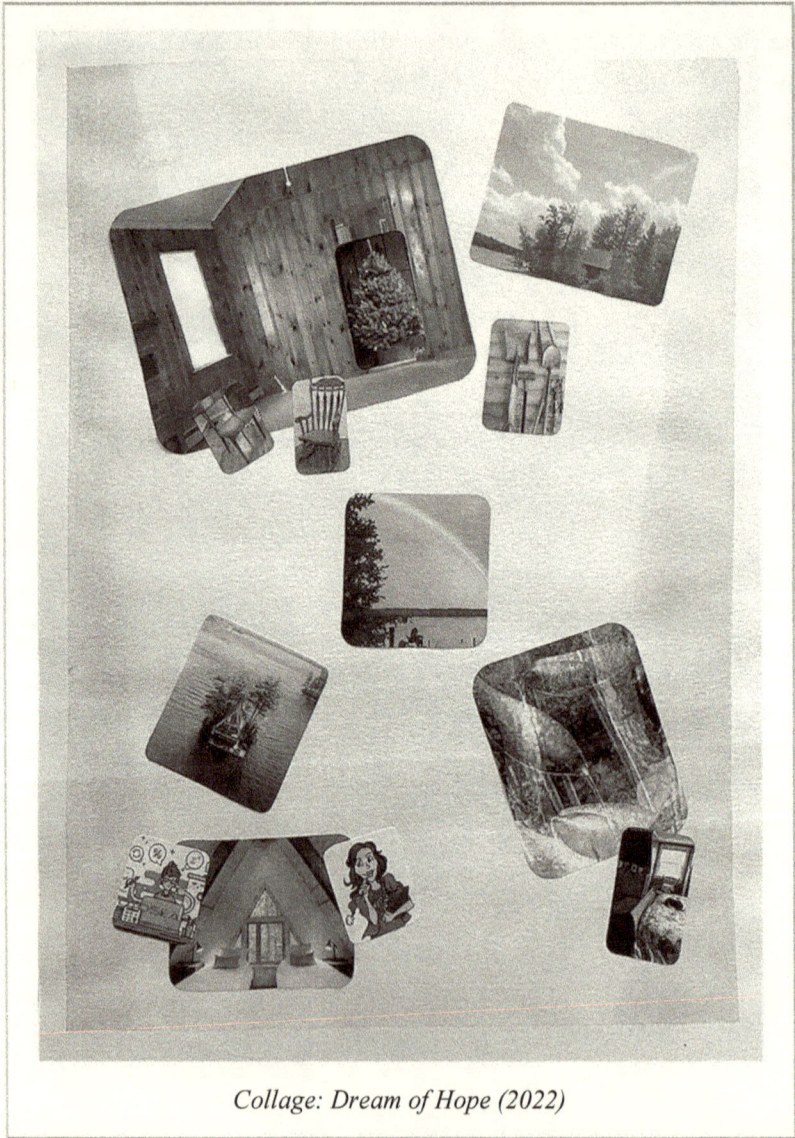

Collage: Dream of Hope (2022)

Tuesday, September 13, 2022

Today, I sold John's car. It was both easy and difficult. I was tired of making sure I drove it at least once a week, keeping up with maintenance, etc.

I received this text from the buyer. I'm crying, in a good way. Yes, I shared John's name with him.

"I lost my father to cancer about 5 years ago. He and I fixed up a similar car just before he died. I sold that car to a 16 year old girl for her first car shortly after his passing. When I drove away today, I saw the same look on your face as I had the day she drove away. It felt like part of him was leaving.

I'm sorry for your loss. Maybe my father, Rick, and your husband met today. Thank you for passing his car on to my daughter. I'd like to know your husband's name in remembrance of him. Thank you very much and God Bless."

Tuesday, September 20, 2022

Today is the third anniversary of John's death. Like the first and second anniversaries, the days and weeks leading up to it have been harder, with more tears, more heartache, than the days in the rest of the year. It's not that every second of every day is filled with grief. It's that the waves, which aren't quite as frequent, are as big as they've always been. I'd heard that's how it is, but couldn't fathom it. Now I know: grief doesn't lessen, I'm now better able to carry it.

This early morning, three years ago, in lucid dreaming, I saw John rise up out of his body on the hospital bed, fully dressed in his signature jeans and flannel shirt, and head towards the front door. When the caretaker called to me to come down NOW, I knew. I held John's hand, cupping his face, as his breathing changed, telling him I loved him and that I'd be OK, he could go, even though I knew he was already gone, his body was just catching up. His breathing was more and more erratic. Then it wasn't. To this day, I don't know if his last breath was in or out, or some odd combination of both.

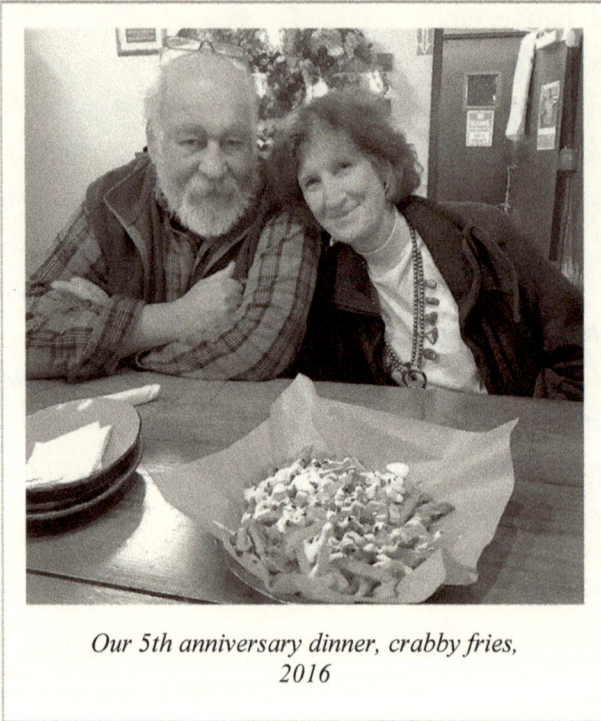

Our 5th anniversary dinner, crabby fries, 2016

Then, six months later, Covid and the isolation that imposed. It was both blessing and curse. I didn't have to pretend I was OK for people who expect grief to be done in six months. Neither did I have the blessing of being with people who knew John, so we could share stories and hold each other in mutual grief. This past spring, like most of us, I began coming out of that isolation. May 28th, my mother died. She was 94 and very ready to go, but still.

I'm changed, deeply changed, by both grief and isolation. There are ways in which I no longer know myself. The ground beneath my feet is unknown. Yes, the externals all appear the same and… the world doesn't seem as bright and I feel purposeless. I'm unsure why I'm still here.

Physical health problems (persistent nerve pain that's finally, after a year and half, being treated, along with insomnia because of pain) haven't helped. I'm aware this can be a powerful place to rest in. I'll make my way through this, with the help of friends, my therapist, and physical therapy. My challenge is asking for the help I need. I'm getting (a little) better at that.

Today, please take a moment to savor and appreciate the very ordinariness of just one of your relationships: with your spouse/significant other, a parent, a child, a good friend. Notice the way that relationship just flows, how breakfast or coffee together just seems to happen, without thought, the almost "back-groundedness" of the relationship. That is what's most precious. That is one thing I've learned these past three years that I didn't truly know before, because it was just there, without question.

Looking Back

I found so much closure in year three, all of it welcome. I understand now why people are encouraged to wait a year before making big decisions like moving, although sometimes they have no choice. Grief brain, which means we cannot think well or clearly, means that making decisions is usually too overwhelming on top of learning how to live with our loss and our grief.

PART XIII:
YEAR FOUR

Friday, September 23, 2022:

> *Kristina: Elmdea you may not remember me but your words and vulnerability make me feel your pain and I am grateful to carry a tiny bit of it.* 🖤🖤🖤
>
> > *Thank you for helping me see and cherish our morning routine in new light.*
> >
> > *I really appreciate it.*
> >
> > *Bless your dear, beautiful, hurting heart.*
> >
> > *May you breathe deep and drink deep and carry on in love and light… and darkness and shadow… and balance.*
>
> *Lili: Dearest Elmdea, thank you for sharing your pain with us. John was such a wonderful gift to us, we are so blessed to have met you both and know him however briefly in the scope of his life. He left his influence which we carry within us… the ripples of a purpose we often aren't conscious of. You are the same. The moments that you come to my mind and heart are moments when I am looking for guidance or inspiration in the shape of tolerance, patience, intelligence, creativity, and warmth. Sending you a long hug and looking forward to our next meeting in person.* 🖤

Friday, October 21, 2022

John's father died today. He was 100. I've so wished I could have known him better, but he and John had a difficult relationship and then, after John's death, Covid got in the way of getting together. May he rest in peace.

Tuesday, October 25, 2022

I lost Miz Alice today. She was John's cat and she adjusted, but she just wasn't quite the same after he died. I'm recovering from Covid, so Joyce took her to the vet for me. I kinda already knew, but didn't want to know, that her time here was done. Joyce said Alice let her know she was tired and ready to go. And John was there to "catch" her as she left her body.

It's soooooo very quiet here now.

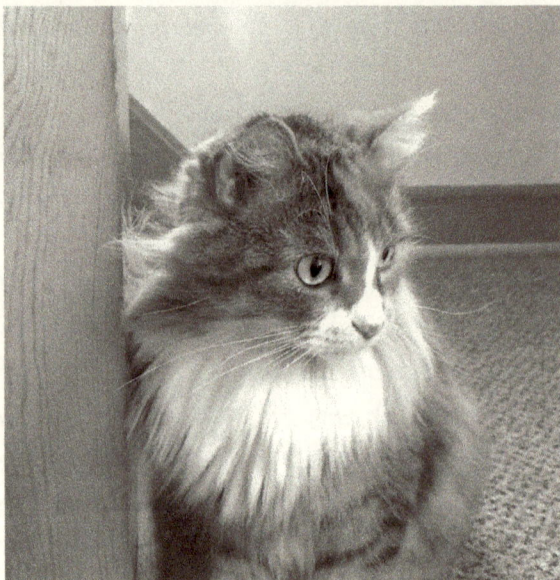

Miz Alice, 2015

* * *

I'm so very tired. It comes and it goes. Some of it is Covid. Some of it is the unrelenting losses: of people (John, my mother, my father-in-law), my health, relationships, now Miz Alice.

I intellectually know it's part of aging. That doesn't mean I like it. I just keep plodding on.

Wednesday, January 18, 2023

I began looking for a house in Winchester today. Over the past year, I've realized this house John and I shared is getting too much for me. For starters: two flights of narrow stairs to do laundry.

I've loved living on the top of a ridge with clear views of sunrises and sunsets, having 4½ acres, so there's privacy. There are also six outbuildings. It's time for someone else to love it. They'll be the third owners of this little farm house built in 1940.

Winchester is really home for me. Berkeley Springs was home when John was alive because John was home.

Tuesday, June 20, 2023

I closed on my house in Winchester today. I made the offer in April and it was accepted, provided I waited until today for closing. It's a ranch built in 1994 with lots of light and well taken care of.

The HOA President is someone I used to work with back in my corporate days. I took that as a good sign and it has been. The interior walls all need to be painted, as do the shutters and garage door. The HOA mandates that we only use Colonial Williamsburg colors on the exterior. Soooo … I wanted purple shutters and garage door. Carter Hall Plum for the win. Not a bright purple, but it is purple.

There are a few other things that need to be taken care of before I move in and, given scheduling of folks, I'm aiming for mid-August, by my birthday.

Saturday, June 24, 2023

I'm in Lewes, Delaware. I came down here on Thursday. Yesterday I got together with some of John's family for a bit.

Today is the triple funeral and burial: John, his father, and his father's partner, Ero.

John's urn has been with his father since the wake on September 28, 2019. Given the pandemic, having a funeral service just didn't make sense. It's been a gift to see so many who knew my John so well, to have some short conversations, to share grief.

This has been easier than I had anticipated. There is a kind of closure. John is buried with his parents. It's not where he wanted to be, but it's where his father, who outlived him, needed him to be. I'm grateful to Mara for getting all of this figured out and arranged. It was no small thing, given she was burying her very beloved mother, Ero.

Sunday, July 9, 2023

Something unusual happened today. I went out to my car to go to the farmer's market. I heard a scrabbling sound coming from underneath it. I stepped a little closer, same sound. Hmmm.

So, wondering what I was getting myself into, I knelt and looked. It was a fawn! It was well under the center of the car and obviously having difficulty figuring out what to do.

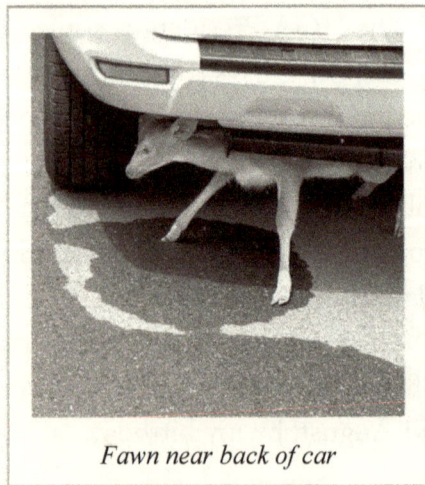

Fawn near back of car

I had zero idea how that little thing was going to get out from under there. There wasn't enough height for it to get on its knees, let alone stand. Yes, it got there but... So, I started talking to it, in a soft

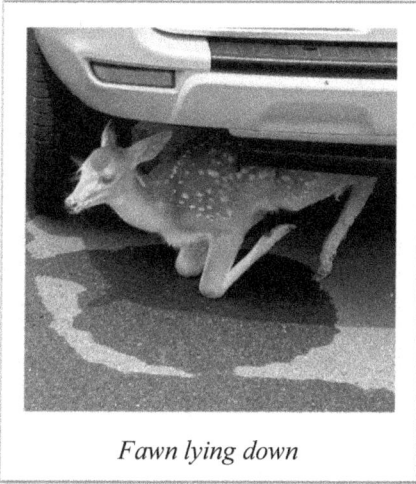

Fawn lying down

voice. "Hi sweetie. Come on out here. It's ok. Come on out here, sweetie." I lightly scratched my fingers against the asphalt. "It's OK. You'll be safe. You can come out this way."

And it did! It crawled/scrabbled towards me, totally trusting. "That's it, sweetie. You can do it." It reached the rear of the car on its poor knees and stopped. It paused, then lay down. We were maybe 3 feet apart, maybe. I told it what a good fawn it was. It lay there, calmly looking at me.

Somewhere in there, I got my phone out of my purse and I took a few photos.

I moved back a little then walked around to the side of the car. The fawn got the rest of the way out from under the car and bounded off towards the woods.

I'm sure mama found it. Or if not mama, one of her herd mates.

I feel so very blessed by this encounter. The utter trust of that little being. I was honored, deeply.

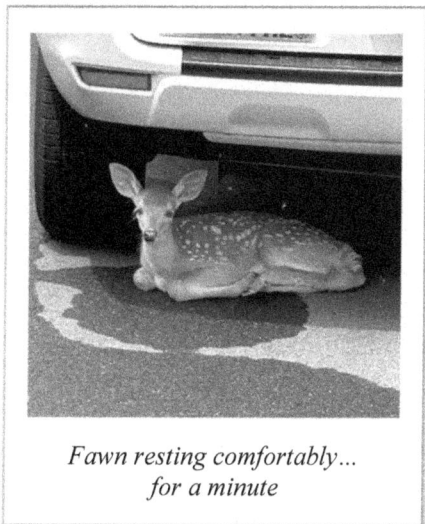

Fawn resting comfortably...
for a minute

Sunday, July 30, 2023

(posted in a private grief group)

I'm so grateful for this group! I don't write much, but I do read a good number of the posts. I'm three years and ten months on this grief journey. I'm now in the process of downsizing so I can move to my new home, in a community with a lot of support.

When my John was alive, he was my home, so it didn't matter where I lived. Now it does. This downsizing though. It's WAY harder than I thought it would be. I keep finding things and the next thing I know I'm crying. Best I can come up with is I'm deconstructing our shared life together here in this house. It would be so much easier to do if he was here... and I doubt we'd be downsizing or moving if he was here. That double bind/paradox thing.

I just miss him. And I'm grateful I can cry and grieve. It feels right and good. It's not as raw. There's a richness to it now, and it still hurts. But y'all know this.

I'm excited about the new house I'm moving to. I'm looking forward to reconnecting with some of my old friends. Not all of them. Some of them don't seem to be interested in being in touch. That's OK. We've all changed in the 14 years since I moved to Berkeley Springs. Other friends get where I've been and how I've changed. They're cheering me on. John isn't here to do that. He was so good at that.

Yup, I'm rambling here. Thank you all of you here. I'm especially grateful right now for those who have recently posted your experiences three plus years out. Your posts have helped me immensely.

Virtual hugs to you all.
#moving

Monday, August 14, 2023

So today begins the final deconstruction of the home John and I created together. There are tears and grief. Yes, it's been 3 years, 11 months and this grief has a new feel to it. Another big letting go. This is hard in a way I hadn't expected. Please think of me over the next few days as I move to Winchester and re-enter/recreate my life there.

Despite it being hard, I've had more signs than I can remember that this IS the right time and right move. It's just the immediate that's hard.

The movers are here, packing up what I'm taking with me. There's a lot that's staying, some from the prior owner, some from John, who collected so many things, and some things of mine. All of that will be auctioned on-line and I'll post that when it's live.

Whewwww!!! This is both hard and exciting.

* * *

Monday, August 14, 2023

> *Laurie: Oh honey. I know just how hard it all is. I had to clean out my parents house 2 years ago. There were tears, confusion, laughter, and some WTF moments sometimes all within 2 minutes 😄 (As someone who has helped me plan steps and organize you would've been super proud). The estate auction for my mother in law this past spring was particularly poignant. It's hard. And it's a process. And yet it's healing. You can do this. 🩶*

Wednesday, September 20, 2023

Today… today is the 4th anniversary of John's death. My grief isn't as raw as it was in the first years. It remains present, as it will until this body draws its last breath. Some days it is front and center, many days it rests quietly in the background.

This is normal grief, folks. Not "complex", not "complicated". Deep grief doesn't "go away in 6 months" as our death denying culture wants us to believe. Life continues, tears arise, deep breathing occurs, new experiences are embraced, grief surges and retreats, we figure out who we are now in this new life without the deeply beloved.

I am well. I'm experiencing moments of pure joy in my new home in Winchester. I'm grateful. I cuddle the bear made from John's favorite polar fleece blanket. The Northern Shenandoah Valley has always felt like home, in a soul-deep way. I'm rediscovering my connections to it, making new friends, reconnecting with old friends.

Life is good.

It isn't what John and I had planned and dreamt. It's what life is: change. I don't know about you, but me and change have a pretty on again/off again relationship. I embrace the idea. The reality is a tad tougher, lol.

Thank you for reading my ramble.

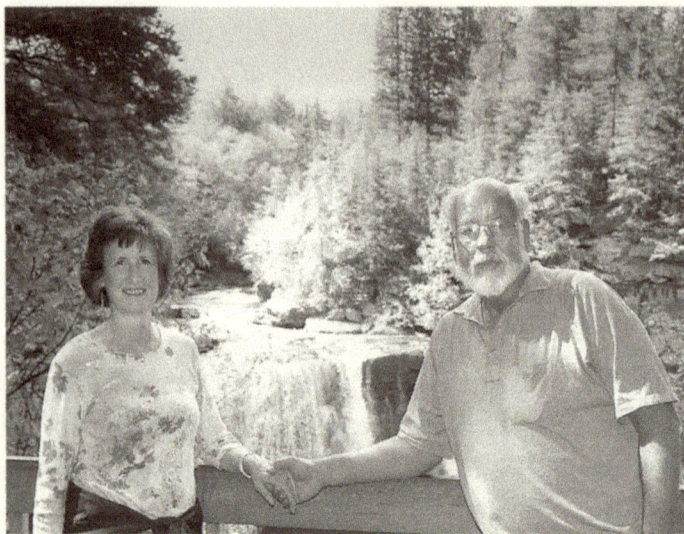

John and me on our honeymoon at Blackwater Falls
May 22, 2011

I miss him, a lot.

Looking Back

I was ready to move back to Winchester long before I was able to do so. In some ways, I was hoping that the move would solve some problems, my isolation in particular. Pandemic isolation and the fear that accompanied it have been difficult for me to undo, but I'm making progress.

My heart is in the Northern Shenandoah Valley. I feel more at home here. I have so many friends here from the years before John and I met. Almost everything I need is a ten minute drive, instead of being an hour one way. I know this town so well. I'm so grateful. I'm so grateful for many things.

The difference in the process of John's death and my mother's death is striking. John still had things he wanted to do, to experience. He worked hard to find peace and grace with the fact that he was dying and he would never do or experience those things. My mother had reached a place where she was ready and at peace.

I can understand that now. If I died in my sleep tonight, I'd be OK. Yes there are things I'd like to do and experience, but they aren't necessary for me to feel I've had a good life. I have. It's a kind of peace with what life is: we're here and then we aren't

PART XIV:
YEAR FIVE

Friday, September 29, 2023

Just two more days on this auction. It starts closing at 7 on Sunday evening.

It's been strange to see all these things, some so very, very familiar, seeming such an integral part of my life and now... not. And knowing it's right for them to go on to their next people. Like a knitted hat I've had for decades and haven't ever worn. But it's been just part of the constant background of my life. Now it won't be.

And then there are other things... things that just came with the house. Being cleared out so the new owners will have a clean slate to start with.

Tuesday, October 17, 2023

The sweet little house that John and I shared is now on the market. It has let me know that "I'm not your house anymore." I've spoken with it and thanked it for its sheltering and caring of John and me. I even hugged it (in an upstairs hall doorway).

It truly doesn't feel like "my house" anymore. It feels like a house, not my home. This is good and proper.

Built in 1940, it's waiting for its 3rd owners. My dream for it is someone who wants a mini homestead with good, dependable wifi. But it may be dreaming of someone else. I trust it's choosing.

Monday, October 23, 2023

I took a walk through the garage on the property in Berkeley

Springs. There were two things. One was a sparrow that had gotten trapped in there. I let it out. The other thing was, way back on a deep shelf was a cardboard box that had been overlooked by everyone. In it were two of John's high school yearbooks and a lot of John's old bills and bank statements. I brought it home and was about to sort through it and toss most of it. Then I stopped. It was a reminder of John's essential messiness. It's now in a slender file box. I can look at it when I want to remember. I doubt there will be any more John messes to clean up.

Friday, November 10, 2023

John's watch is still running. It's losing time, but it's still running, four years, one month, and 21 days after his spirit left his body and that body took its last breath. It's a metaphor for my grief. My grief has changed. Unlike the watch, which will stop one day, my grief will remain with me the rest of my life. Because that's what deep grief does. It's an intrinsic part of me now. And that is right and proper.

It's about love.

Monday, December 4, 2023

This past week has been extraordinary. I was up at the old house three times.

A week ago Sunday, I was just checking things out, adjusting the thermostat, turning off lights. Walking out to the last porch/attached garage, I noticed a whole snake skin, from tail to head. It was a good 3 feet long, a black snake. I love those snakes. Among other things, they eat mice. Yes! The skin felt like a gift from the house.

I was up again on Monday, after seeing Margi. There were some outlets without covers so I put those on and I put on some of the colorful, fun switch plates that used to be up there. I'd thought they'd work in my new place, but they don't. The really special thing? There was an old deer skull with horns sitting in the driveway. It was a two year old buck, with one antler shorter than the other. It felt like another gift from the house. It's now resting on a bed of dried sage in my new home.

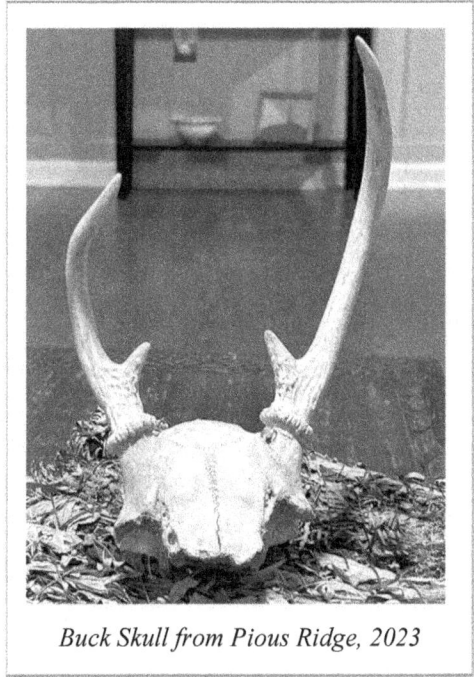

Buck Skull from Pious Ridge, 2023

On Wednesday, I had a cash offer on the house. Way lower than I wanted. I was with Anne and Sally for our writer's group and, for some reason, I just lost it and started crying. It was all kinds of loss. It didn't make sense, but it didn't have to. It felt good to just cry. Then Sally shared how much she had enjoyed John's company and his stories. It's one of the few times since he died that someone has shared their memories and experiences of and with John. Her memories re-awakened my own memories of him as he was before he got sick. I'm so very grateful.

My realtor made a counter offer and, eventually, we all agreed on a selling price, with a closing date on or before December 20!

Then I heard back from my potential editor for this book, saying she'd like to work on it with me and offering some suggestions that already have me excited.

So many good things, all in one week. I'm grateful.

This house I'm now living in is feeling more and more like home. I've no interest anymore in living in the old house. None. It's done. I've moved forward with my life.

This meme showed up years ago. It's the best visualization I've found of what grief really is. My grief hasn't gotten smaller, I have grown around my grief. I will continue to do so. I'm grateful.

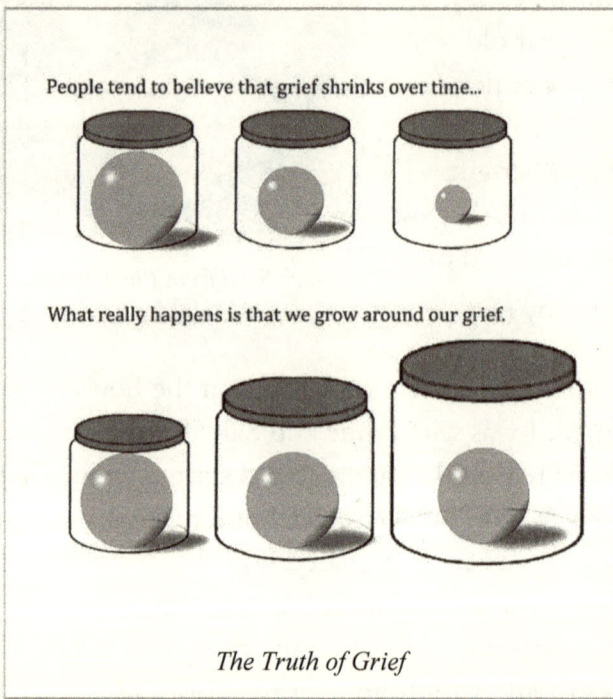

People tend to believe that grief shrinks over time...

What really happens is that we grow around our grief.

The Truth of Grief

Monday, February 5, 2024

It's official. The house John and I lived in closed today. It belongs to someone else whose first name happens to be John. I'm relieved I'm not responsible for it any more. It was too much: 4 ½ acres with six outbuildings on a ridge top with amazing sunrises and sunsets. The sort of place so many of us dream of.

Here's the REALLY interesting thing: Cindy, my realtor and friend, stopped by with a lovely car blanket, which is her "congratulations, your house is sold" gift.

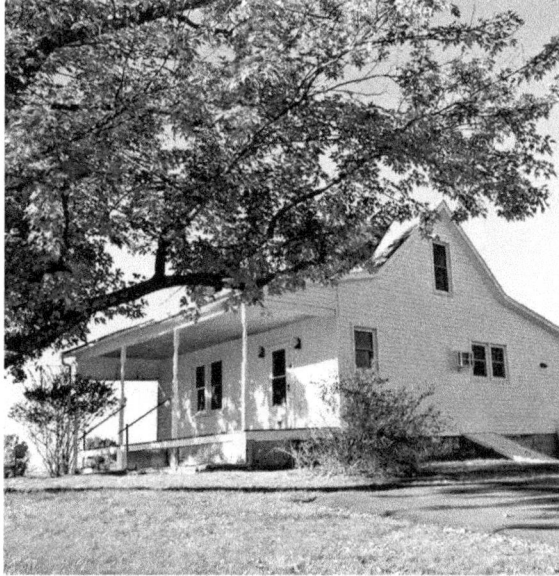

Our West Virginia House,
Realtor photo

She also brought a bouquet of roses. She said she kept getting a sense that John wanted her to buy me flowers. She never knew John. I started crying.

What she couldn't know was John used to buy me flowers every other week or so. It feels like he wanted to let me know he's celebrating the sale of the house too. In the last months of his life, he wanted the house fixed up so I could live there for the rest of my life. I told him I couldn't promise I would. Today, he let me know he's good with my choice to sell the house we shared.

I suspect I'll grieve the house and the memories I could physically touch there. Part of this larger, longer process of missing him… that is my companion.

Here are his roses, via Cindy as his delivery angel.

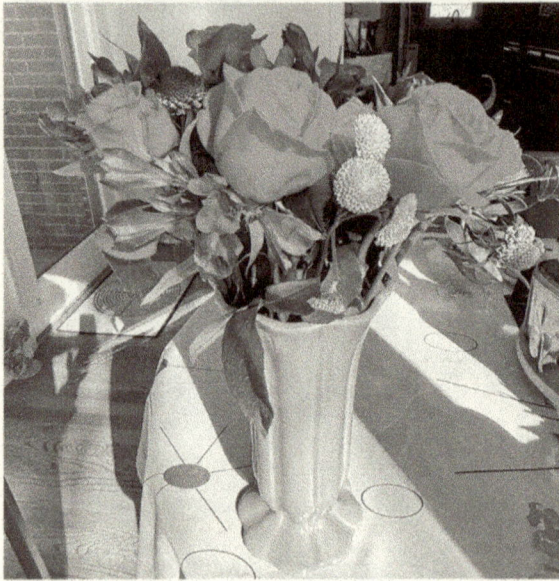

Congratulatory Bouquet from John, 2024

Sunday, June 23, 2024

It's been a year since we all gathered in Lewes to bury John, his father, and Ero. Today, Mara shared a pic of John's memorial marker. It's beautiful, with its two sprigs of Salvia on it... sage, just as he was. Seeing those dates caught my attention. I have a relationship with those dates. I've never felt a relationship with dates on a tombstone before. There is a kind of closure, a sort of peace, that I hadn't anticipated. I love you, dear one. I love you.

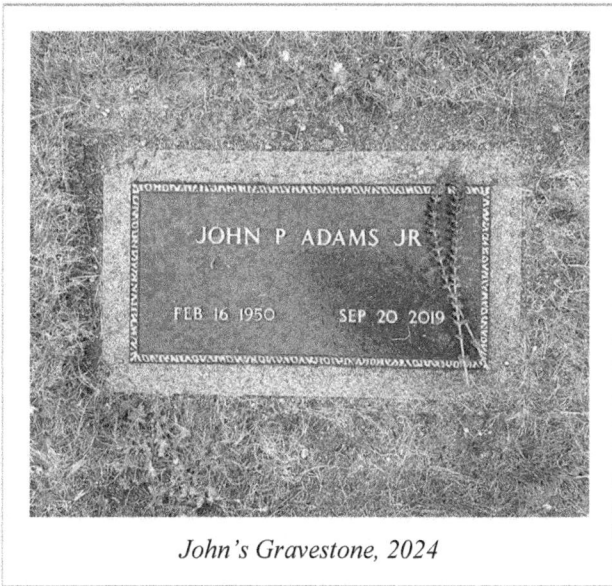

John's Gravestone, 2024

Looking Back

Moving back to Winchester was the right choice. Much as I miss the Ridge, with its trees, critters, and memories, being in town is where I need to be now. The snakeskin and the deer skull are treasured final gifts from the land that John and I cared for and loved for fourteen years.

I'm grateful there's a small herd of deer that graze, and sometimes nap, in my new yard throughout the year. Yes, they browse on my shrubs. I'm still grateful they're here. There isn't much wildlife in town so I deeply appreciate those who are here.

Very importantly, John hasn't given me any flak for burying him in Lewes with his parents, even though he'd told me years before that he didn't want to be buried there. He never said where he *did* want to be buried, so I chose what I felt was best for the living, particularly his father, who had lost his only child, as well as the rest of John's family. He and his father had resolved their father/son issues in the two visits they had after John's diagnosis. I also knew that John's perspective was much different after his death.

PART XV:
MOVING FORWARD

Friday, September 20, 2024

Today marks the 5th anniversary of John's death. I've purposely kept today clear, with no appointments or things to do.

This year is a tad easier than the past anniversaries. Why? Because I had a visitation from John about a month ago. He's appeared in a few dreams, but it never felt never like this. It felt like he was actually in the room with me. If you think about it, you'll know what I mean, how you not only see and hear someone in a room with you, you sense them as well. It was that kind of feeling. I haven't felt his physical presence for 5 years. It was unmistakable and unlooked for.

I had gone to sleep the night before, asking for the answer to a question in dreamtime. I asked that it be clear and easily remembered. When I woke up the next morning, there was no memory of anything.

It was then that I felt John behind me. In my inner ear, I heard him say "You need to eat." It was pure John. When I was having a bad day, he used to ask me "Did you eat breakfast today?" My answer was usually "No. I forgot." His saying that I need to eat confirmed it wasn't my imagination.

I still cry sometimes. I continue to miss him. I'll always wish he were here. I'm soooo very grateful we had the years together we did. We both wanted more, but that wasn't the way it worked out.

I hope I have more visitations and I know they are rare. This one has granted me great peace. We had agreed, before he died, that he would let me know if he still existed after his death. He does. While I've known he does, it was more intellectual, a belief. Now? Now I know. Thank you, John. I love you 🖤🖤🖤

Tuesday, August 12, 2025

John visited me again a few weeks back. I was at The Monroe Institute for their Discovery program, listening to one of the exercises. During the third section of the music, I physically felt hands coming from behind my chair and resting on my arms. I "knew" it was John. I hadn't been expecting, asking, or looking for a connection with him. We had an ordinary sort of conversation, so ordinary I still don't remember exactly what we spoke about, just that it was comforting to have that sort of conversation with him again. As we spoke, I could tell that he's been growing over there, just as I have here. It's a beautiful thing that we continue to grow together, each in our way, in our own places. I was in tears, good tears, loving tears. Weeks later, I still know exactly where his hands gently rested on and held my arms.

The sixth anniversary of his death is a little over a month away. I feel peace. Yes, I still mourn and I am moving forward in unexpected ways, creating a new website, getting out with friends more, volunteering, and taking better care of myself. I'm finding purpose again.

And now, this book truly is complete.

* * *

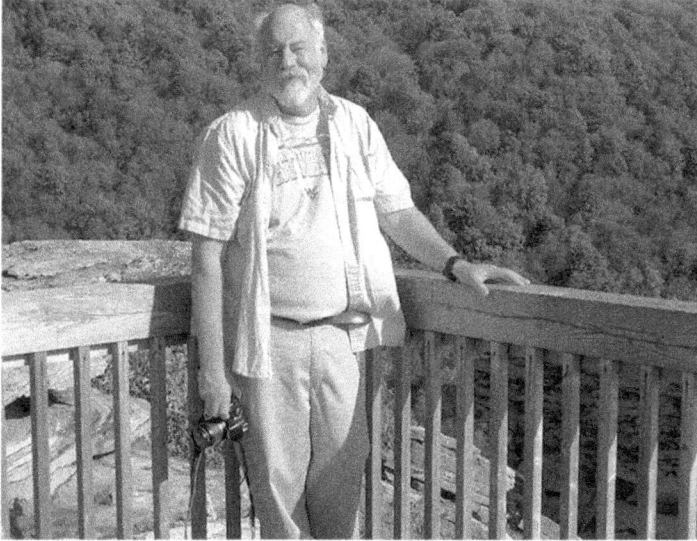

John, during our honeymoon at Blackwater Falls
May, 2011

It is a strange thing, to be subject to both love and death.

Especially when neither can prevent the other.

— Martha Brockenbrough
The Game of Love and Death

* * *

PART XVI:
CLOSING THOUGHTS

I'll always wonder about not getting a second opinion. To be clear, I don't feel guilty that I didn't push for one. John was adamant he wanted to go to the University of Maryland Marlene and Stewart Greenebaum Comprehensive Cancer Center (UMGCCC). He had researched his options and found they were among the best in the country for esophageal cancer. Further, he already had a referral to UMGCCC from the gastroenterologist at UMMC who had worked with him earlier. I did everything I could to support John's choices about his treatments and when to stop them. Finding the path that honored his wishes while also advocating for him with him was an ongoing process. While I would have made different choices, it wasn't about my life. It was about his life and his soul's journey. I'm forever honored I was blessed to walk the last eight years of his life with him. They were the best years of my life.

Odd as it may sound, I'm grateful John didn't have deal with me dying first. I think it would have been harder for him. In talking with other widows, many of us feel the same: grateful our beloveds have been spared this grief.

Completing this memoir has been deep work for me. As I wrote, and as you've read, there were many times I thought the manuscript was complete and I could handle reading all my caretaking posts and journal entries to begin editing. I couldn't. I needed more time, more than the two years I initially thought I'd need. This book has been an ongoing reminder that grief has its own timeline, for each of us.

The first time I was able to read this book from beginning to end was a few months before it was published and five years, seven months (there will always be counting) after John's death.

That was when Lyn, my wonderful and supportive editor, sent her final edits (mostly punctuation, paragraph breaks, and the like) for me to review. I made a few final changes and additions and it was finally, truly, complete.

My other struggle has been sharing so much that's so very personal, despite knowing that the experience of deep grief is universal and we deep grievers understand each other, often from a place that comes from before words. Despite being an introvert and very private person, I felt compelled to gather my posts and entries together as an offering to my fellow cancer caregivers and grievers.

At its core, the creation of this book is about being of service. I hope it will be helpful and supportive to you and to your family and friends as they support you.

I have glimmers of my purpose going forward. While not necessarily connected, I'm a volunteer with Hospice, with a food co-op, and perhaps a local museum. I knit a lot. I read a lot. I've begun editing a fantasy novel I wrote, then set aside, eleven years ago. I know there will be surprises, because there always are. Life does that.

* * *

If you are a caretaker or if you're looking at end of life options for yourself, I invite you to contact your nearest hospice and see what services they offer, both for caretakers and the dying. Hospice care can give an increased quality of life.

While I initially complained that they created more work for me, it was absolutely worth it. To sign up with Hospice, you need to be considered within 6 months of dying. I've heard stories of folks who graduated from Hospice and lived for another 6 months or even years. You never know. The comfort they provide, both physically and emotionally, is beyond price.

Their end-of-life counseling helped John find peace and grace. Their grief counseling kept me sane while I was caring for John and after he died.

I'm forever grateful to The Hospice of the Panhandle (HotP) in Kearneysville, West Virginia. The Hospice services we received were free because HotP is a non-profit and billed Medicare. I strongly recommend finding a similar non-profit Hospice. Most insurance does accept billing from Hospice.

* * *

In closing, I invite you to treasure the ordinary,
everyday moments
you share with your beloveds:
morning coffee, yard work, sitting on the porch,
fixing dinner, talking things through, quick hugs…
My memories of those ordinary moments are what sustain and
comfort me.

PART XVII: LIFE PIRATE

(A short story)

Author's Note: While character's names and the type of cancer have been changed, this is based on several real experiences, as told to the author.

* * *

The Pirate

Beautiful seas right now, such rich reds and pale yellows!

Another awareness trickled into my consciousness, a new area for exploration and plundering. Yes!

I've had an extraordinary life: well-fed, ever-expanding horizons, always growing. My first memories are hearing my host as she read stories of pirates, swash and buckle. She read other stories, called "history," "biography," "fantasy." Those were sort of interesting, but they didn't resemble my life much. The books she called "space opera" were fun. But the ones called "pirate books" are the best because that's what I am, a full-blooded, full-bodied pirate.

Over the past bit of time, which gets kinda fluid here, I've been feeling the pull to explore again. My ship is sturdy and strong, with lustrous planks. My fins navigate the red and yellow seas. I know, pirate ships in the stories have sails, but there's no wind on my seas. There are very strong currents and no horizons. So, fins it is. My fins are half-opened, gleaming fans of pastel yellow, their surface is embroidered with delicate red lines, the same red as the seas we swim.

Have I mentioned I have a magical ship? I discovered this a bit ago. I'd been exploring when a land mass appeared, so I explored it for booty. It was ripe for pillaging and setting up an outpost. That's when the magic happened.

One of my planks disengaged, floated to the island, and firmly attached itself to a small rise just off the shore. It was a most natural thing, even though I hadn't done it before. My awareness expanded the instant the plank became an outpost. That plank grew and thrived, just like me, exactly like me. The plank touched the island. It grew into an outpost.

There are six outposts now. We talk to each other all the time. I hadn't realized I was lonely for my own kind until that first outpost established itself. That drove me to search for more welcoming islands. My host's stories are interesting, but my outposts are lots more fun.

Then today, something happened. An assault, a horrid assault. A colorless foreign substance invaded my seas. It's eating away at my beautiful ship, at my outpost's ships. It hurts… a lot!

The Friend

Anthea sat in mediation, breathing in, breathing out, again, again. Her friend, Sarah, had just been diagnosed with gallbladder cancer. The long-term prognosis was six to twelve months, with chemotherapy. Radiation and surgery would have to wait until the chemo shrank the tumor.

An unfamiliar presence made itself known as she sat. Continuing to breathe, Anthea just watched, to see what, if anything, developed.

It's Sarah's cancer! No. It couldn't be. Yet it is. Hmmm. It's a living being, with a kind of consciousness. I wonder if I can talk to it?

Anthea's shoulders relaxed as she sat more firmly on her purple meditation cushion.

I see you. Anthea sent the thought to the presence. She sensed a response.

She explored the presence more. Its only focus was growing and expanding. She nodded. Yes, that's what cancer did. It ignored the cell death messages that routinely happened in the human body.

"This may be a dumb idea, but there's nothing to lose."

Anthea spoke aloud, needing to hear the words as the idea formed in her mind. "I'll send it compassion and information instead of anger, hatred, and battle."

Dear cancer, I know you are only doing what you know how to do. You are doing it beautifully. What you need to know is that you will die. There is no way around it. What you have is a choice about how you die. If you keep colonizing, you'll end up killing Sarah, your host, and you'll die because your colonies will eat her up and she'll die. Sarah is doing something now called chemotherapy. Those drugs are to kill you off bit by bit until you are greatly diminished. Then there will be something called radiation, which will burn you, followed by surgery, which will cut you out of the body you are living in. Your choices, from what I can see, are to ignore me and continue to grow, which will kill both you and Sarah, or let go and allow the chemotherapy and radiation to diminish you so when the surgery happens, it will be easy for you to detach from her. It's your choice.

The Pirate

My name is cancer? I didn't know that. I'm killing my host? My teller of pirate stories? My source of food and outposts? What I heard has rattled everything I know about myself.

I'll consider this later.

Now others are speaking to me, saying the same things that first person did, the one who isn't my host. I don't understand how I can "hear" them. What I do know is they speak with different tones and colors than my host does. They all say they honor me and how dedicated I have been living the only life I know. They go on to say, yes, I will die. My only choice is how. I need to be with this for a bit. Meanwhile, one of my older outposts just said there's a new territory that looks promising. Do I go?

The Patient

The nausea. I hadn't believed it could be this bad. My friends warned me, but I had hoped to avoid all of that. A constant state of nausea. Almost, but not quite, feeling like I need to throw up, an almost constant tightness and lump at the bottom of my throat.

And I'm tired. My feet have gained weight, or my shoes have. They weigh at least fifty pounds each. It doesn't matter which shoes I wear. Walking from one room to another is a day's exercise.

The oncologist had said food would taste weird. Ummm, yeah. Like gasoline, or like it's gone moldy, or like bitter chemicals. But I have to eat. The medical marijuana helps some, but not enough. This isn't the way I had planned to lose weight.

Losing my hair was anticlimactic. The strange part was the tingles and near-itches on my scalp. That's what dying hair follicles feel like. My hats and my wig are easier to manage than even the thought of the energy I used to put into washing and drying my hair. I shaved it when it started tingling. I was sooooo not interested in discovering clumps of it all over the place.

The fear is the worst. I do my best, but there are so many new sensations and feelings in my body I don't know what's important and what isn't. It doesn't help that I can't think straight. Thinking wears me out, it's so hard some days. "Chemo-brain" is a real thing. This chemo / radiation / surgery program has to work. I've got things I still want to do with my life.

I have so many books on my Kindle waiting for me. But I can't focus enough to remember the last sentence I read. I remember reading my first book all the way through when I was in first grade. I love exploring other places, the way authors think and create.

I've wanted to write since I was a kid, but I never felt like I knew enough. I'm rethinking that now. But when I open my laptop to start typing, the words get all jumbled. I can barely type coherent things on my Facebook timeline, let alone answer everyone's questions about how I'm doing. I appreciate their concern and their love. I really do. Heart emojis are my new best friend.

What I miss even more than reading is being outside for hours on end. Smelling air that unabashedly proclaims Spring. It's the same with the light. Spring light is totally different from Autumn light. Maybe it's the angle of the sun or something. I'd like to find out why that is.

The colors, the unfoldings, the sheer exuberance of nature in the spring. Last year, there was a forsythia clinging to a steep road embankment. The flowers were a waterfall of yellow down the bank. The soft magenta of redbud, the clear pinks of cherry, the white of dogwood, the complexities of greens as trees leafed out, grasses started growing. All of it. I wish I had painted it last year. I've always painted, but I was too self-critical. Now? Now just to hold a brush, mix colors, and let my heart lead my hand, instead of over-thinking like I usually did. Life really is too short to mess with anything that isn't love.

I'm watching Glenn do his best to take care of things. He has always been good at organizing, unlike me. If there's an empty space on a table or a counter, it's there to put something on. If there isn't any empty space, no problem, I'll just pile whatever it is on top of something else. Glenn's being so patient with me and giving me more leeway than he used to. Glenn is a wonderful cook. I wish I could actually eat some of it. I daydream of eating his Thai food. These days, I'm all about protein shakes and ice cream. Something that goes down easy and has half a chance of staying down. Spices aren't my friends any more.

This cancer has its own ideas and life. I'm going to give Althea's suggestion a go. It can't hurt. Battling this cancer hasn't been fun at all, at all. And it doesn't seem to have helped either.

The Husband

Anthea stopped by a few days ago and shared this crazy idea: talking to the cancer, having compassion for it. That's the last thing I feel. If it had a neck, I'd wring it and stuff it down the garbage disposal. Even that would be too kind.

I feel so helpless. There's so little I can do. Making doctor's appointments and driving Sarah there, keeping track of her meds, getting them refilled, ordering her protein drinks, taking out the trash, mowing the yard, and I'm not sure what else. Those are easy, no big deal. But there's nothing I can DO about the cancer and what it's doing to her.

My Sarah, the Sarah I know and love, isn't around much these days. Instead, I see a stranger in her body. It makes sense, when I think about it. She's focused on doing what she can to encourage healing while dealing with nausea and all the other side effects of that chemo. At the same time she's staring death in the face.

I wasn't happy about her decision to do chemo. It's so destructive, so beyond awful, what it does to the body. And it's not my life. I don't know what her soul's journey and purpose is. I have to trust, a lot. There are moments when it's easy, like when we get to laugh at something and she's present, here again, even for a few moments.

I'm alone in a way I've never felt alone before. There's no one I know who understands what I'm going through, what Sarah's going through, how little can be done except hope. This loneliness is not about Sarah's introspection. It's a new place inside me. An emptiness that echoes nothing.

One day at a time. That's all I can do. If I look too far forward, I can see a life without Sarah. I'm not ready for that. I never will be. And I'll talk to that cancer. It can't hurt. What did Anthea say? I don't have to like it, but I can feel compassion for it. It's a stretch, but I'll do it because Sarah has asked me to.

The Pirate

I was made to grow and expand and feed. But I'm pirating the life of my host. I've always known she was my host. It never occurred to me I wasn't good for her, or bad for her. I was alive. She was alive. Together, we lived.

My outposts aren't much help right now. They think exactly like me because they are me. My host tells me she loves me, but she wants to live. To stop growing and colonizing is against my nature; it's my only purpose. I don't know how to do otherwise.

I'm being eaten alive by these foreign invaders and I hurt. My host is getting weaker, so more areas are opening up, but the invaders kill every plank that goes out to colonize.

I thought I was the captain, but now I know she is. Since I'm to die, I'll do it in style. I lack a cutlass and pistol so I'll maroon myself by letting go of all my outpost islands. This is one time when marooning is honorable. My host has been good to me, giving me everything I needed to thrive and grow, sharing all the booty. Now I must be good to my host.

There. It is done.

All of us are now adrift. We'll be swept away. It's a proper payment for our good life.

The Patient

"Sarah? Can you hear me? The operation went well."

It's hard work finding my place in the world, in my body, in my mind. Oh, yes, general anesthesia. That explains it. I hear her voice again.

"Sarah? It's Dr. Krane. It's okay. The operation went well. You're coming up out of anesthesia."

Somewhere I remember how to nod my head. I speak. "Cold." The comforting weight of a warmed blanket settles around me like magic.

The third time my mind comes back up, the doctor is still here, or here again. Glenn is here too. He's holding my hand I think.

Dr. Krane. I've liked her from the beginning. I'm glad she was my surgeon.

"I've done a lot of these operations, Sarah. This one was different. It was like that tumor wanted to come out, like it wanted to let go. It detached so easily. You're a lucky woman."

Yes, I am. I am going to paint, and read, and love Glenn, and write, and twirl in the sunlit air.

PART XVIII:
RESOURCES

Books that helped me the most

(I've marked * the two I most strongly recommend you purchase for yourself if you need to pick)

Callanan, Maggie and Patricia Kelley, *Final Gifts: Understanding the Special Awareness, Needs, and Communications of the Dying*, 1992, Bantam Book, New York, NY

* Cornwall, Deborah J., *Things I Wish I'd Known: Cancer Caregivers Speak Out*, 2016, Bardolf & Company, Sarasota, FL

* Devine, Megan, *It's OK that You're Not OK*, 2017, Sounds True, Louisville, CO

Devine, Megan, *How to Carry What Can't Be Fixed*, 2021, Sounds True, Louisville, CO

Hagar, E. M., *A Hospice Chaplain's Field Guide to Caregiving*, 2019, Zip Sisters Publishing

Anticipatory Grief

Grace, J. C., *Anticipatory Grief Daily Journal*, 2016, CreateSpace Independent Publishing Platform

Hodgson, Harriet and Lois E. Krahn, *Smiling Through Your Tears: Anticipating Grief*, 2004, BookSurge, LLC, North Charleston, NC

Biographies/Memoirs

Alexander, Elizabeth, *The Light of the World, A Memoir*, 2015, Grand Central Publishing, New York, NY

Bauerschmidt, Tim, and Ramie Liddle, *Driving Miss Norma: One Family's Journey Saying "Yes" To Living*, 2017, Harper One, New York, NY

Kalanithi, Paul, *When Breath Becomes Air: What Makes Life Worth Living in the Face of Death*, 2016, Vintage, London, UK

Kubler-Ross, Elisabeth, MC, *The Wheel of Life, A Memoir of Living and Dying*, 1997, Touchstone, New York, NY

Riggs, Nina, *The Bright Hour: A Memoir of Living and Dying*, 2017, Simon & Schuster, New York, NY

Shannon, George, and Chad Patrick Shannon, *The Best Seven Years of My Life: The Story of an Unlikely Caregiver*, 2018, George B. Shannon

Cancer

Mukherjee, Siddhartha, *The Emperor of All Maladies: A Biography of Cancer*, 2010, Scribner, New York, NY

Turner, Kelly A., *Radical Remission, Surviving Cancer Against All Odds*, 2014, Harper Collins, New York, NY

Caregiving

American Cancer Society, *Cancer Caregiving A to Z: An At-Home Guide for Patients and Families*, 2008, American Cancer Society, Atlanta, GA

Bucher, Julia A., ed., and Peter S. Houts, ed. and Terri Ades, ed., *Complete Guide to Family Caregiving: The Essential Guide to Cancer Caregiving at Home*, 2011, American Cancer Society, Atlanta, GA

Menard, Ellen, *The Not So Patient Advocate: How to Get the Health Care You Need Without Fear or Frustration*, 2009, Bardolf & Company, Sarasota, FL

End of Life

CommonPractice.com, *Hello: The Conversation Game for Living and Dying Well*, Elkins Park, PA

Gawande, Atul, *Being Mortal: Medicine and What Matters in the End*, 2014, Penguin, New York, NY

Keeley, Maureen P. and Julie M. Yingling, *Final Conversations: Helping the Living and the Dying Talk to Each Other*, 2007, VanderWyk & Burhham, Acton, MA

Kessler, David, *Visions, Trips, and Crowded Rooms: Who and What You See Before You Die*, 2011, Hay House, Carlsbad, CA

Kubler-Ross, Elisabeth, MD, *Death is of Vital Importance: On Life, Death, and Life After Death*, 1995, Station Hill Press, Barrytown, NY

Miller, B. J., and Shoshana Berger, *A Beginner's Guide to the End: Practical Advice for Living Life and Facing Death*, 2019, Simon & Schuster, New York, NY

Puri, Sunita, *That Good Night: Life and Medicine in the Eleventh Hour*, 2019, Viking, New York, NY

Smartt, Lisa, *Words at the Threshold: What We Say As We're Nearing Death*, 2017, New World Library, Novato, CA

St. Pierre, Joellyn, *The Art of Death Midwifery: An Introduction and Beginner's Guide*, BookSurge, Virginia Beach, VA

Grief

Derman, Deborah S., *Colors of Loss and Healing: An Adult Coloring Book for Getting Through Tough Times*, 2016, Rodale Press, New York, NY

Didion, Joan, *The Year of Magical Thinking*, 2006, Vintage International, New York, NY

Dintino, Susan, *Grief Reliefs, A Companion for Your Grief Journey*, 34 Card Self-Care Oracle Deck, 2019, https://griefreliefs.com/

Greene, Jayson, *Once More We Saw Stars, A Memoir*, 2019, Alfred A. Knopf, New York, NY

Hickman, Martha Whitmore, *Healing after Loss: Daily Meditations for Working Through Grief*, 1994, William Morrow, New York, NY

Hughes, Kristoffer, *The Journey into Spirit, A Pagan's Perspective on Death, Dying, and Bereavement*, 2014, Llewellyn Publications, Woodbury, MN

Kennedy, Alexandra, *Honoring Grief: Creating A Space To Let Yourself Heal*, 2014, New Harbinger Publications, Oakland, CA

Kessler, David, *Finding Meaning: The Sixth Stage of Grief*, 2019, Scribner, New York, NY

Kubler-Ross, Elizabeth and David Kessler, *On Grief & Grieving: Finding the Meaning of Grief Through the Five Stages of Loss*, 2005, Scribner, New York, NY

Leder, Steve, *More Beautiful Than Before, How Suffering Transforms Us*, 2017, Hay House, Carlsbad, CA

Lewis, C. S., *A Grief Observed*, 1961, Harper Collins, New York, NY

Rea, Rashani, and Francis Weller, *The Threshold Between Loss and Revelation*, 2017, Sacred Spiral Press, Na'alehu, HI

Weller, Francis, *Entering the Healing Ground: Grief, Ritual and the Soul of the World*, 2012, WisdomBridge Press, Santa Rosa, CA

Weller, Francis and Michael Lerner, *The Wild Edge of Sorrow: Rituals of Renewal and the Sacred Work of Grief*, 2015, North Atlantic Books, Berkeley, CA

Websites/Blogs

Bereaved People Aren't Strong, We're Trying To Survive:
https://johnpavlovitz.com/2020/01/04/bereaved-people-arent-strong-were-trying-to-surviving/

Coping With Grief During the Holidays:
https://experiencelife.com/article/coping-with-grief-during-the-holidays/

Grief
https://grief.com/ (David Kessler)

Grief and Holidays: What the Bereaved Need From Friends and Family: https://thelifeididntchoose.com/2016/09/03/grief-and-holidayswhat-the-bereaved-need-from-friends-and-family/

Holding Space:
https://heatherplett.com/2015/03/hold-space

How Grief Changes the Brain:
https://www.psychologytoday.com/us/blog/widows-walk/202208/how-grief-changes-the-brain

Newly Widowed Checklist:
https://thelizlogelinfoundation.org/resources/newly-widowed-checklist/

Refuge In Grief:
https://refugeingrief.com
https://refugeingrief.com/videos/how-to-help-a-grieving-friend-the-animation

ACKNOWLEDGEMENTS

Anne Larsen and Sally Brinkman – Sometime in 2012 or 2013 our writer's group began. We've met mostly every couple of weeks since then. You're my dear friends and you've helped me become a better writer. I deeply appreciate the way we bring our particular strengths and knowledge to our critiques of each other's writing. IMHO, our writing group is the best ever.

Cindy Burdette – your grief counseling when I was caretaking John and continuing after his death helped me find my way in a world that had changed beyond recognition.

Margi Griffiths – Your counseling and friendship over the course of six years helped me discover who I am now.

Lyn Worthen – your feedback and suggestions as my editor and book birther allowed me to set aside my overwhelm about how much editing and revision this memoir would need. That was the final piece I needed to fully embrace and complete it.

Susan Lyon – my dear friend of fifty plus years, you know me so well, as I know you. You've helped me regain my footing time and again. We have great laughs and deep understanding.

* * *

ABOUT THE AUTHOR

Born in Boulder, Colorado, Elmdea spent her childhood exploring the hills and old mining roads just outside her backdoor, seven miles up Four Mile Canyon. When she wasn't doing that, she was far, far away in as many books as the old library would let her check out at one time.

She began writing when she was nine: a simple short story. Over the years, she has written journals, poetry, procedures manuals (somebody had to), short stories, non-fiction, and a still-developing fantasy novel.

In her late forties, a health crisis propelled Elmdea to do some deep soul searching. As a direct result, she resigned from her Fortune 500 middle management position and became a certified Past Life Regression Therapist.

Elmdea is the author of Moving Forward, The Journey of a Cancer Caregiver; Stories of Past Life Healing (the 2nd Edition of Liberating Incarnations: Twenty-Five Stories of Past Life Regression); and short stories that have been published in multiple anthologies.

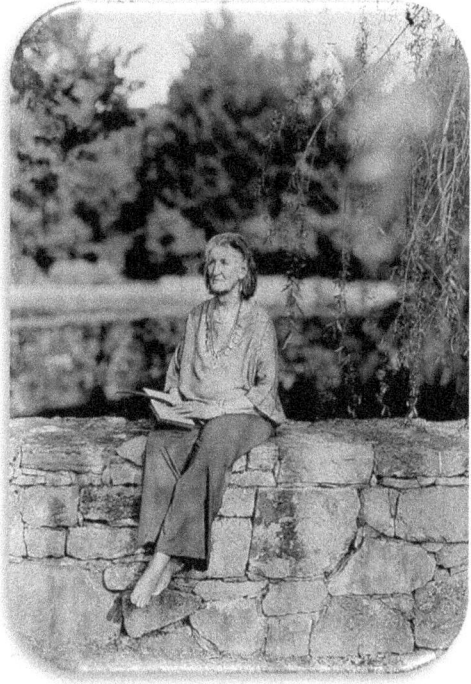

Now gratefully retired, Elmdea continues to write and finds knitting to be a meditative practice. She misses the skilled editorial assistance of Miz Alice, her late beloved kitty.

For more information, visit www.ElmdeaAdams.com

* * *

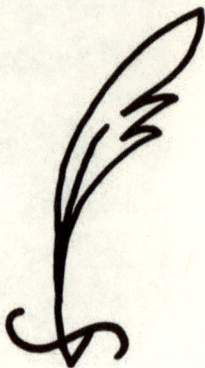

www.ingramcontent.com/pod-product-compliance
Lightning Source LLC
Chambersburg PA
CBHW031940080426
42735CB00007B/206